Immunology

Other books in the Biomedical Sciences Explained Series

0 7506 3256 9   Biochemistry *J.C. Blackstock*
0 7506 2879 0   Biological Foundations *N. Lawes*
0 7506 3254 2   Biology of Disease *W. Gilmore*
0 7506 3111 2   Cellular Pathology *D.J. Cook*
0 7506 2878 2   Clinical Biochemistry *R. Luxton*
0 7506 2457 4   Haematology *C.J. Pallister*
0 340 76374 4   Human Genetics *A. Gardner, R.T. Howell and T. Davies*
0 7506 3467 7   Medical Physics *J. Trowbridge*
0 7506 3253 4   Molecular Genetics *J. Hancock*
0 7506 3415 4   Transfusion Science *J. Overfield, M. Dawson and D. Hamer*

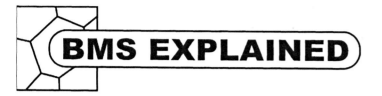

Immunology

B. M. Hannigan BA(Mod) PhD FIBMS
Dean, Faculty of Science, University of Ulster, Coleraine, UK

Series Editor:
C. J. Pallister PhD MSc FIBMS CBiol MIBiol CHSM
Principal Lecturer in Haematology, Department of Biological and Biomedical Sciences,
University of the West of England, Bristol, UK

A member of the Hodder Headline Group
LONDON
Co-published in the United States of America by
Oxford University Press Inc., New York

First published in Great Britain in 2000 by
Arnold, a member of the Hodder Headline Group,
338 Euston Road, London NW1 3BH

http://www.arnoldpublishers.com

Co-published in the USA by
Oxford University Press Inc.,
198 Madison Avenue, New York, NY 10016
Oxford is a registered trademark of Oxford University Press

Whilst the advice and information in this book are believed to be true and
accurate at the date of going to press, neither the authors nor the publisher
can accept any legal responsibility or liability for any errors or omissions
that may be made. In particular (but without limiting the generality of the
preceding disclaimer) every effort has been made to check drug dosages;
however, it is still possible that errors have been missed. Furthermore,
dosage schedules are constantly being revised and new side-effects
recognized. For these reasons the reader is strongly urged to consult the
drug companies' printed instructions before administering any of the drugs
recommended in this book.

British Library Cataloguing in Publication Data
A catalogue record for this book is available from the British Library

Library of Congress Cataloging-in-Publication Data
A catalog record for this book is available from the Library of Congress

ISBN 0 340 76381 7
1006124654

1 2 3 4 5 6 7 8 9 10

Typeset by David Gregson Associates, Beccles, Suffolk

What do you think about this book? Or any other Arnold title?
Please send your comments to feedback.arnold@hodder.co.uk

Contents

Preface

Immunology is a young, exciting and dynamic science which developed as a specialist aspect of other Biomedical Science disciplines: cell biology, biochemistry, haematology, microbiology and pathology. New knowledge in immunology and immunology-based biological tools are now enabling further development of those other subject areas. The biotechnology industry that is revolutionizing our lives owes much of its existence to research in immunology.

An understanding of fundamental concepts in immunology and of its applications is an important part of Biomedical Science education. This text aims to make your learning as easy as possible. The further reading that is recommended includes 'popular science' books. How can you be afraid of a science that so many non-scientists choose to read about?

The internet is a valuable source of immunology information. Many web-sites excel in providing up-to-date databases that allow the learner or researcher to find the information they need. Immunology is indebted to advances in bioinformatics that enable access to resources such as sequences of genes and proteins that influence immune responses. You won't find individual web-site addresses in this book – they change too frequently. But fortunately there is Biomednet (www.Biomednet.com). Go there, follow directions, and you'll find all the internet immunology resources you'll need.

I enjoyed writing this book, but could never have completed it without the secretarial skills and support of Caroline Adams and the talent and professionalism of Mark Miller and Killian McDaid in the Faculty of Science Cartography office. Thank you all.

B. Hannigan

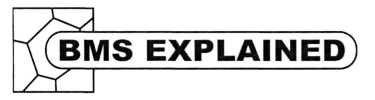

Series preface

The many disciplines that constitute the field of Biomedical Sciences have long provided excitement and challenge both for practitioners and for those who lead their education. This has never been truer than now as we face the challenges of a new millennium. The exponential growth in biomedical enquiry and knowledge seen in recent years has been mirrored in the education and training of biomedical scientists. The burgeoning of modular BSc (Hons) Biomedical Sciences degrees and the adoption of graduate-only entry by the Institute of Biomedical Science and the Council for Professions Supplementary to Medicine have been important drivers of change.

The broad range of subject matter encompassed by the Biomedical Sciences has led to the design of modular BSc (Hons) Biomedical Sciences degrees that facilitate wider undergraduate choice and permit some degree of specialization. There is a much greater emphasis on self-directed learning and understanding of learning outcomes than hitherto.

Against this background, the large, expensive standard texts designed for single subject specialization over the duration of the degree and beyond, are much less useful for the modern student of Biomedical Sciences. Instead, there is a clear need for a series of short, affordable, introductory texts, which assume little prior knowledge and which are written in an accessible style. The *Biomedical Sciences Explained* series is designed specifically to meet this need.

Each book in the series is designed to meet the needs of a level 1 or 2 student and will have the following distinctive features:

- written by experienced academics in the Biomedical Sciences in a student-friendly and accessible style, with the trend towards student-centred and life-long learning firmly in mind;
- each chapter opens with a set of defined learning objectives and closes with self-assessment questions which check that the learning objectives have been met;
- aids to understanding such as potted histories of important scientists, descriptions of seminal experiments and background information appear as sideboxes;
- extensively illustrated with line diagrams, charts and tables wherever appropriate;
- use of unnecessary jargon is avoided. New terms are explained, either in the text or as sideboxes;
- written in an explanatory rather than a didactic style, emphasizing conceptual understanding rather than rote learning.

I sincerely hope that you find these books as helpful in your studies as they have been designed to be. Good luck and have fun!

C.J. Pallister

Acknowledgements

To Bill, Ben and Ross – my family.

Chapter 1
The immune response explained

Learning objectives

After studying this chapter you should confidently be able to:

State the overall function of immune responses.

State the two principal types of immune response.

Discuss the evolution of immune responses.

Describe the location of the immune system within the human body.

What is immunology?

Immunology is the study of how the human body can remain intact and unharmed in the midst of a vast universe of other life-forms and inanimate objects which might otherwise threaten our survival. It is an exciting and rapidly changing subject within the Biomedical Sciences.

Since the evolution of multicellularity it has become necessary for each organism to contain cells and molecules capable of defending it. These cells and molecules comprise the **immune system**. Through immunology, students, clinicians and researchers can discover the components of the immune system, how it functions and how communication can take place between the immune system and the rest of the body which is being protected. Our current understanding is of a complex but highly organized immune system; indeed, as in many aspects of science, the more we learn the more clearly the organization becomes apparent.

So, the **immune system** is a series of cells, some organized as discrete components within tissues, and molecules which work together to allow immune responses to occur. All of the important components are in place but in a non-responsive or resting state until the person, the host, is exposed to something that they must be defended against. Thus the function of immune responses may be stated as:

to provide protection against anything that would be harmful to the host

Not everything that the host comes in contact with is potentially harmful, so the immune system must be able to 'decide' when to mount a response. The decision to respond or not to respond is, without doubt, one of the most critical functions of the immune system and it has proved extremely difficult for scientists to reach agreement on how this decision is made. The state of non-responsiveness is known as **immunological tolerance**, i.e. the opposite of response. Indeed, at the beginning of the twenty-first century, just over a century since the first useful application of immunology, many aspects of the debate have not yet been resolved and we are left with a number of conflicting hypotheses. Immunologists are now seeking to design experiments which will test their hypotheses. From all of the ideas currently prevailing it is necessary to select a working model through which students can begin to understand at least the central concepts. It is through questioning of such models that many great strides in understanding may be made.

It is useful to have a generic name that can be used to refer to all things that may be the targets of immune responses. Targets may be:

- infectious organisms (bacteria, viruses, fungi, yeasts, parasites);
- macromolecules (foods, drugs or chemicals);
- cells (tumour cells or cells in mis-matched transfusions or transplants).

The collective term most commonly used is '**non-self**', i.e. whatever is not part of the host, or '**self**'. Further definitions of 'non-self' and consideration of mechanisms by which the immune system decides what is non-self will be fundamental to later chapters.

What types of immune response occur?

The most basic type of defence is that provided by the body's **physical and chemical barriers**. These barriers are present in the presence or absence of non-self so they involve little or no element of 'response'. The barriers regulate the initial interactions between host and non-self and so exist at the **interfaces** between the individual and the environment. It must be remembered that the environment is not just external but also internal. At the external interface skin, tears and sweat are effective physical and chemical barriers to non-self; tears and sweat contain anti-bacterial substances, most notably the enzyme lysozyme in tears and the normal bacterial flora of the skin. At the point where the internal environment meets the host the range of defences is greater, including:

- the acid pH of the stomach (neutralizes ingested bacteria);
- normal bacterial flora of the intestine (inhibits growth of pathogenic bacteria);

- mucous membranes (inhibit microbial invasion into tissues);
- mucus transport and cilia which line the gastrointestinal, respiratory and genito–urinary tracts (aids the removal of bacteria from body systems).

Humans are able to exert some control over both their internal and external environments. Externally, we use disinfectants and antiseptics which reduce the numbers of microorganisms; for the same purpose we practise good hygiene and we have an innate sense which allows us to avoid contact with potentially harmful substances, physical injuries or sources of infection. Internally, we again try to reduce the load of microorganisms by taking antibiotic or antiviral drugs and we try to avoid consuming foodstuffs or beverages that would be harmful, either through their chemical nature or the presence of contamination. We also try to avoid the introduction of potential hazards into other internal spaces by, for example, avoiding unsafe sexual practices with potentially infected partners or not inhaling apparently noxious fumes. It is interesting to note that the total external surface area over which host and non-self can interact is many times smaller than that of the internal interface. The total adult skin surface is some 2 square metres while there are some 400 square metres of mucosal surface including the gut, respiratory and genito–urinary tracts. It is vital that our internal interfaces are well-defended.

Despite the obvious effectiveness of physical barriers, they are routinely overcome. For example, cuts or abrasions to the skin, whether occurring accidentally or deliberately such as during surgery, permit non-self to enter host tissues. The elimination of gut bacteria through antibiotic overuse allows potentially harmful bacteria to colonize the gut and lesions of the gastrointestinal tract wall permit microorganisms that normally would be excreted to enter the tissues. It is when non-self has breached the physical barriers that the body normally begins to mount an immune response.

The first wave of responses constitutes 'natural' immune responses for which the collective term **acute inflammation** is commonly used (Chapter 3). It is important to remember that these rapid inflammatory responses are intended to be beneficial. In later chapters instances will be presented of inflammation that is associated with pathological situations; long-lasting **chronic inflammation** (Chapter 7). However, an acute inflammatory response which takes place in an appropriate position and is resolved at the appropriate time, is not harmful. The principal features of natural responses is that they are:

- inborn;
- unchanging;
- non-specific.

This means that, provided the individual is healthy and not immunosuppressed in any way, natural immune responses are always the same regardless of the type of non-self which is being targeted.

Acute inflammation is a highly effective process which results in the elimination of many otherwise hazardous forms of non-self. However it is not sufficient to endow the individual with any long-term benefits. A useful analogy of an organism which has only natural responses in its defensive arsenal is a person who attends school every day of his or her life from age 5 to 25 but who is unable to remember any of what he or she learns. This person would then have to be re-exposed to exactly the same information in each of her 20 years of schooling and would emerge no more competent than on day 1. This is obviously wasteful and contrary to biological systems which we know to undergo constant adaptation and change in order to cope better with their environment. The immune system is no exception and mammals have evolved **acquired, or adaptive, immune responses** (Chapter 5). The key features of acquired responses are memory and specificity.

Memory causes the immune system to be permanently altered on every encounter with non-self. **Specificity** allows each response to be tailored so as to be the most appropriate for dealing with the particular type of non-self being confronted at a particular point in time or location. So, learning, in the context of the immune system, means acquiring the ability to respond with greater efficiency each time the system is called upon to deal with non-self.

Acquired immune responses are further sub-divided into **cell-mediated responses** and **antibody-mediated responses**.

Antibody-mediated immune responses are sometimes termed 'humoral' responses. This name reflects the archaic term 'humor' which meant a body fluid. Antibodies were originally described purely as soluble proteins within the fluid phases of the circulation, i.e. lymph or blood plasma.

Can we track the evolution of immune responses?

At the beginning of the twentieth century the work of two great pioneers of immunology was recognized with the award of the 1908 Nobel Prize in Medicine to Elie Metchnikoff and Paul Ehrlich. Many other Nobel Prizes have been won by immunologists since that time and you will find details of their achievements peppered throughout the chapters of this book. Quite a lot of early work was done on very simple animal species. Even the simplest animals need to provide a defence against all other components of their environments.

Alongside the knowledge that animals possessed a defence system made up of cells and molecules came the realization that this power had been present in simple creatures such as starfish since the time they originally evolved, some 600 million years ago. Elements of the human immune system that we know today are detectable in virtually all living organisms. The subject known as comparative immunology allows us to study how the immune system differs in different species. By observing what aspects of immune responses are present in simple animals, we conclude that those responses are of the most ancient origin. Responses that are possible only in higher animals, such as mammals, probably evolved more recently.

Many invertebrates can produce only natural responses, thus the acquired response is probably of more recent origin. Clearly, however, the ability to recognize non-self is well-developed. Some of the very simplest creatures, for example protozoans such as paramoecium, consist of only a single cell. Nonetheless, that one cell can defend itself in a way that is remarkably similar to **phagocytosis** by specialized immune cells in the human (Chapter 3). Multicellular animals of increasing complexity gradually diversified their immune responses. Phagocytic cells are present in invertebrates together with the ability to produce soluble mediators that resemble the **cytokines** of higher animals (Chapter 3). These soluble mediators ensure that communication takes place between different components of an animal so that defences can be appropriate, effective and initiated when required. Cytotoxic cells are present in animals such as sponges, corals and annelids (earthworms). In general, the comparatively simple defence system of each species of lower animal must be sufficient to deal with the potential threats to that species. Further additions were made to the 'arsenal' of the immune system thereby increasing the complexity of responses. New components added to the system included both a range of immune cell types and a great diversity of molecules. The molecules are present both as components of cells, especially the outer cell surfaces (Chapter 4), and as molecules secreted into extracellular fluids and the circulatory systems. In mammalian immune systems large families of molecules have been discovered that bear structural, and/or functional similarities to other members of their family. For example, the **immunoglobulin gene superfamily** comprises molecules that participate in immune responses and are found predominantly on cell surfaces. It is thought that such families arose through gene duplication events and subsequent mutation of each family member.

The pattern of changes that led to the evolution of mammalian immune systems may well have been spurred by changes in the environment. One such change is thought to have been the evolution of warm-bloodedness which allowed bacteria and other microorganisms to proliferate more rapidly within their hosts. The hosts which survived to reproduce were those that were best able to halt the growth of their aspiring colonists, i.e. those with the most effective immune responses. At that time point it is likely that **germinal centres** evolved in a number of tissues throughout the body. Germinal centres permit rapid increases in the number of immune cells to occur when the cells are needed.

The principal structural feature that characterizes members of the immunoglobulin gene superfamily is a sequence of approximately 110 amino acid residues known as an immunoglobulin domain. The secondary structure of the domain includes disulphide bridges.

Where is the immune response located?

There is quite a simple answer to this question which, as time passes, looks more and more correct. The answer is that the immune system is everywhere in the body. Yes, of course, there are specialized cells and molecules which are the only ones able to carry out particular functions but the actions of these special cells cannot take place in isolation. There must be constant cross-talk and interaction between these cells and other cells and tissues throughout the body. In particular, the immune cells must be able to exchange messages with components of the other major regulatory systems: the brain, nervous systems and endocrine system. An idea that the circulatory systems, i.e. the blood, lymph and tissue fluids, are the major site of immune responses is certainly not appropriate. These circulatory systems are vital, however they are more appropriately regarded as transport systems ensuring that cells and molecules can reach their correct destinations. The most significant responses take place within tissues. In the past few years immunologists have begun to understand the cellular and molecular features which actually allow, indeed encourage, the immune cells to leave the circulation and enter the tissues in response to a variety of stimuli. For this reason the **vascular endothelial cells** that line the blood and lymphatic vessels may be considered to be key regulators of immune and inflammatory responses (Chapter 3). They provide a dynamic interface between tissues and the circulating fluids, cells and molecules.

Immune responses may contribute to disease processes

Under certain circumstances the responses generated by the immune system may cause harm to the body. Sometimes, for example, when responses are directed against infectious microorganisms, damage to normal healthy cells may occur (Chapter 6). So the disease processes that we observe when infectious organisms are present may not all be caused directly by the organisms but rather by the body's response to the organism. Other responses may be excessively strong, for example in the case of hypersensitivities, e.g. allergy (Chapter 7). Our current understanding of the range of diseases known as **autoimmune diseases** would suggest that defects may occur in the immune system that lead it to destroy parts of the host itself, e.g. in rheumatoid arthritis, multiple sclerosis or diabetes (Chapter 8).

Despite these severe, and sometimes fatal, consequences of immune responses, nature has provided us with some unfortunate examples of how difficult it is to survive in the absence of a functional immune system. One or more components of the immune system may be defective or absent in **immunodeficiency** diseases (Chapter 9). People with these conditions suffer recurrent infections. The types of infection depend on which component of the immune system is defective. Some deficiencies may be so severe that the person dies from overwhelming infection. If a baby is born with a severe immune deficiency, death from infection is likely to occur before the second birthday. Our observations on people infected with the **human immunodeficiency virus (HIV)** show clearly how a progressive decline in immune function goes hand-in-hand with an increasing burden of infections and other diseases such as specific cancers and dementia. The ultimate destruction of the immune system by the virus leads to **acquired immune deficiency syndrome, or AIDS**, which is fatal.

How do we learn more about immunology?

Amazing advances in the scope and understanding of immunology have taken place in the past three decades. However, immunology has a longer history than this, as shown in Table 1.1.

Table 1.1 *Some significant discoveries in immunology*

Year	Person or country	Discovery
3000 BC to 100 AD	Greece, Rome, Far East, Middle East	Disease transmission and immunity Immunization
1798	Edward Jenner	Immunization
1880s to 1890s	Robert Koch	Rational identification of organisms causing infectious diseases Type IV hypersensitivity
	Elie Metchnikoff	Phagocytosis Cellular immunity
	Louis Pasteur	Active immunization
1890s	Emil von Behring	Antibodies
	Paul Ehrlich	Antibody formation
1895–1910	G.H.F. Nuttall	Antisera for diagnosis
1900–1910	Jules Bordet	Complement
	Theobald Smith	Transplacental transmission of antibodies
1900–1930	Karl Landsteiner	Antigen–antibody reactions Blood groups
1945–1955	Peter Medawar	Graft rejection/tolerance
1945–1980	George Snell	Genetics of histocompatibility
1950–1980	Neils K. Jerne	Immune regulation
1959	F. Macfarlane Burnet	Clonal selection theory
1960s	Rodney Porter, Gerald Edelman	Structure–function relationships in antibodies
1974	R.M. Zinkernagel, P.C. Doherty	MHC restriction
1975	G. Milstein, G. Kohler	Monoclonal antibodies
1980s	S. Tonegawa	T-cell receptor for antigen

Information on immune responses can be generated through several of the different traditional biomedical disciplines: biochemistry, haematology and histopathology in particular. Advances in each of these disciplines accelerates the rate of production of new information about immune responses in human health and disease.

How can a knowledge of immunology be applied?

Knowledge of immune systems has revolutionized ideas on many aspects of the aetiology, pathogenesis, diagnosis and treatment of a wide range of human diseases (Chapter 10). This last area, the manipulation of immune responses, or components of the immune system to provide novel treatments for human diseases (termed immunotechnology), is only now beginning to be explored. There have been some initial disappointments where products failed to live up to their apparent potential, e.g. the use of **interferons** or **monoclonal antibodies to treat cancer** successfully. Nonetheless, it is clear that the failures should be viewed as being relative only to the excessively optimistic initial hopes that were based upon incomplete understanding of the processes involved. There is a great deal more immunology that we have yet to discover. There is even more that has yet to be applied.

Suggested further reading

Abbas, A.K., Lichtman, A.H. and Pober, J.S. (1997) Cellular and Molecular Immunology. Pennsylvania: W.B. Saunders.

Davies, H. (1997) Introductory Immunobiology. London: Chapman and Hall.

Gowans, J.L. (1996) The lymphocyte – a disgraceful gap in medical knowledge. *Immunology Today* **17**, 288–291.

Heatley, E.V. (1994) Gastrointestinal and Hepatic Immunology. Cambridge: Cambridge University Press.

Hughes, A.L. and Yeager, M. (1997) Molecular evolution of the vertebrate immune system. *Bioessays* **19**, 777–786.

Ridley, M. (1999) Genome. London: Fourth Estate.

Sharon, J. (1998) Basic Immunology. Pennsylvania: Williams and Wilkins.

Self-assessment questions

1. Distinguish between acute and chronic inflammation.
2. List three ways in which natural immune responses differ from acquired responses.
3. What is the opposite of immunological tolerance?

4. State one type of defence mechanism that is present in simple, unicellular animals.
5. In mammals, what cell type regulates interactions between tissue cells and cells in the circulation?
6. What are the likely consequences for an individual born with an immune deficiency?
7. What are autoimmune diseases?
8. What do 'HIV' and 'AIDS' stand for?
9. How do people with AIDS usually die?
10. What contribution to the development of immunology was made by Edward Jenner?

Key Concepts and Facts

Immune Responses

- Immune responses provide protection against anything that might be harmful to the host, or 'self'.

- Natural immune responses are inborn, unchanging and non-specific.

- Acquired, or adaptive, responses display memory and specificity.

- Acquired responses include both cell-mediated and antibody-mediated immune responses.

Evolution of Immune Responses

- All animals display some element of an immune system.

- Even the simplest immune systems provide the protection necessary for the host.

- Invertebrates mount only natural immune responses.

- The evolution of warm-bloodedness was a spur to the development of more efficient immune responses.

The Human Immune System

- All parts of the body contribute to its defence and an effective communication system is essential.

- The immune system comprises specialized immune cells and soluble molecules.

- Immune responses may cause damage to the host.

- Immune deficiencies lead to multiple infections in the host.

Chapter 2
Components of the human immune system

Learning objectives

After studying this chapter you should confidently be able to:

Describe the organization of the lymphoid system.

Discuss the origins of cells of the immune system.

Describe the characteristic appearance of cells of the immune system under light microscopy.

Explain the different roles of primary and secondary lymphoid tissues.

List the principal non-cellular components of the immune system.

Explain the roles of cytokines.

The human body (the **self**) exists in the company of internal and external spaces. These spaces comprise environments that contain (the **non-self**) organisms and other non-living entities capable of interacting with the self. Specialized cellular structures provide interfaces between the self and the non-self in each space. The interfaces include **barriers** that prevent invasion of the body by non-self. These are the body's first line of defence.

We know that many types of non-self are able to overcome the body's barriers so we need to have tissues, cells and non-cellular factors that provide protection through **immune responses**. Some responses against non-self can be initiated right underneath the barrier layer so our idea of defences being located at interfaces between host and non-self becomes a theme that is carried through to explain the location of many components of our immune system.

Cells, tissues and organs of the lymphatic system

The basic histological organization of the immune system within the body may not be immediately evident because of the apparently scattered nature of its various components. Nonetheless, our current understanding of the many cells and molecules that are involved in immune responses and our ability to distinguish them within tissue or body fluid samples allows us to discern a strategically well-organized system. The **lymphatic system** includes most of the tissues, organs, connecting vessels and circulating cells that are important for mounting immune responses. The tissues of the lymphatic system are known as **lymphoid tissues** and the interconnecting vessels are the **lymphatics**.

The lymphoid system is closely associated with the cardiovascular system and the pathways of the major lymphatics parallel those of the veins. These two systems are intimately linked; the lymphatics transport tissue fluid, known as **lymph**, which originated as the liquid plasma of the bloodstream. Plasma moves from arteries into tissues under the influence of hydrostatic pressure (blood pressure) from the heart. It is important that fluid does not accumulate in the tissues so it is returned to the blood circulation in the principal lymphatic, the **thoracic duct**, when it drains into the right **subclavian vein**. Lymph flow is exceedingly slow compared to that of the blood because it is remote from the 'pumping' action of the heart. Situated along the lymphatics, in a manner often likened to beads on a string, we find the **lymph nodes**. Figure 2.1 shows the main sites of lymph nodes in the human body. Although nodes are associated with all of the main lymphatics they are found clustered especially in the neck, thorax, axilla (armpit), abdomen and groin. The structure and function of lymph nodes is considered further later in this chapter. Lymph nodes comprise just one example of a lymphoid tissue. Figure 2.1 also shows the location of the principal lymphoid tissues (a) in an adult and (b) in a child. It is important to note the differences between these two figures.

All of the important cells and non-cellular components of the immune system spend at least part of their lifespan circulating in the bloodstream. This is the reason why the cells are often called, somewhat mistakenly, blood cells, and the non-cellular components are called blood proteins. The immune cells are distinguished from the most abundant cells of the bloodstream, the red blood cells, by being called **white blood cells** or **leukocytes**. Table 2.1 shows the normal number of cells of each leukocyte type within the peripheral blood. Remember that both the absolute and the relative numbers of different cell types will vary from one body fluid or tissue to another. As blood is the most accessible of all tissues cell counting is routinely performed on blood samples.

The developing immune system

The foetus does not have an independent immune system as it is so intimately linked to its mother. Of course the foetus is foreign to the mother because of its inheritance from the father. Yet the mother's

Figure 2.1 *The principal lymphoid tissues found in (a) an adult and (b) a child. Primary lymphoid tissues have the darker shading. Note that the locations where these occur are fewer in the adult than in the child*

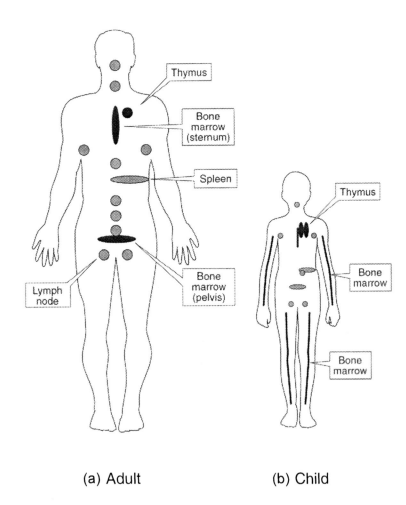

(a) Adult   (b) Child

Table 2.1 *Numbers of different leukocytes in blood*

Cell type	Normal range per mL blood	% of total leukocytes
Erythrocytes	Male: $4.2-5.4 \times 10^6$	
	Female: $3.6-5.0 \times 10^6$	
Platelets	$1.5-4.0 \times 10^5$	
Leukocytes (total)	$5.0-10.0 \times 10^3$	
Neutrophils	$3.0-6.0 \times 10^3$	60
Eosinophils	$50.0-300.0$	1–2
Basophils	50.0	1
Lymphocytes	$1.25-3.50 \times 10^3$	25–35
Monocytes	$0.30-0.60 \times 10^3$	6

immune system does not, normally, regard the foetus as non-self so it is not rejected. This everyday miracle cannot yet be satisfactorily explained, although its possible mechanisms are explored in greater depth in Chapter 5. The easier thing to understand is why the foetus does not reject the mother: the foetus has only the smallest beginning of an immune system. It is not until after birth that it really becomes capable of mounting responses. At this stage the child is known as a **neonate**. The earliest site of production of immune cells is the liver which, after birth, loses this function and the **bone marrow** takes over. In the neonate **haematopoietically** active bone marrow is found in the central cavities of many bones, including the long bones of the upper and lower limbs (Figure 2.1b). As the child grows this bone marrow function will decline such that, by about the time of puberty, active bone marrow is present only in the pelvis and sternum (breast-bone). In adults the marrow cavities of long bones are filled with adipose (fatty) tissue.

Haematopoietically active bone marrow contains **stem cells,** termed pluripotential or totipotential stem cells. These stem cells have proved to be very difficult to study and scientists have many unanswered questions about them. Things that we do know about pluripotential stem cells are that they are necessary for the production of blood cells of all types and that they have a self-maintenance and self-renewal capacity that allows them to persist throughout adult life. Unfortunately, the mechanisms underlying stem cell renewal and mechanisms to prevent exhaustion of stem cells are largely unknown. The long-lived haematopoietic stem cells are usually quiescent, their entry into the cell cycle usually being induced only in the presence of a variety of different known and unknown or poorly characterized non-cellular factors. This is probably a safeguard mechanism preventing an exhaustion of the stem cells through excess differentiation, for example, during chronic infections when immune responses are active for prolonged periods.

Haematopoietic stem cells are quite rare and constitute approximately 4–400 in 10^5 normal bone marrow cells. They in turn produce other stem cells each of which can give rise to a more restricted range of blood cells. For this reason such cells are called committed cells or, for historical reasons, colony-forming units. Progress is currently being made towards understanding the factors which regulate each state in the differentiation pathway of white blood cells. One important question that has not yet been answered is 'What stimulates the bone marrow to produce each different leukocyte type?'.

Figure 2.2 shows that cells originating from bone marrow stem cells undergo **differentiation** and **proliferation**. Each differentiation event allows cells to acquire new functions and characteristics. These events are arranged into distinct pathways and each pathway leads ultimately to a particular white blood cell type. Moving along a pathway, or lineage, the cells progressively display the features characteristic of the mature cells of the appropriate lineage and lose their capacity for self-renewal. One cell lineage derives from erythroid stem cells. Eventually these will produce **red blood cells** or **erythrocytes**. Although all tissues in the body are

It would be of great benefit to researchers to be able to isolate functional pluripotential stem cells and to provide them with appropriate stimuli. The cells could then be used to reconstitute damaged immune systems, for example of patients with AIDS, through production of balanced numbers of the different leukocytes. These processes depend critically on the maintenance of a functional haematopoietic microenvironment and the presence of a plethora of non-cellular factors (haematopoietic growth factors). Recent progress has been made to define the molecular basis of how haematopoietic cells become committed to a particular differentiation pathway.

Figure 2.2 *Developmental pathways of blood cells. Each pathway is initiated by stem cells within the bone marrow. Each cell type undergoes differentiation and proliferation to produce mature cells that enter the circulation*

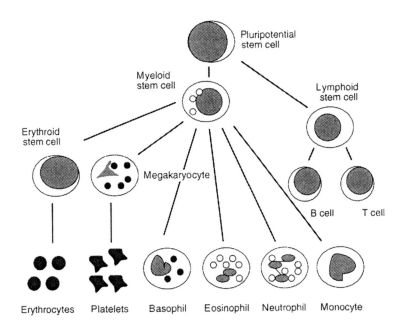

critically dependent on erythrocytes to supply oxygen and remove carbon dioxide, these cells are not considered to form part of the immune system. Also deriving from the bone marrow are mega-karyocytes which produce blood **platelets**. Platelets play significant roles in promoting and controlling blood clotting, or haemostasis. When the body has sustained physical damage haemostasis is essential. It is now clear that this should be considered as part of the body's defence and this concept is strengthened by the fact that platelet products and other components of the blood clotting mechanism interact in many significant ways with the immune system.

Approximately 10^9 nucleated cells are produced per kilogram of body weight within the haematopoietic system per day. Blood loss and cell losses, caused, for example, by a variety of disease processes, infections, or treatment with cytotoxic (cell killing) drugs, can be compensated by an increase in the generation of new cells. This process is called induced haematopoiesis. Increased production of cells is largely restricted to the specific cell type that is required in the particular stress situation: haemolysis (destruction of erythrocytes), for example, induces cells of the erythroid lineage. The lifespan of the fully differentiated mature forms of blood cells may vary considerably, from several hours for some cells (e.g. neutrophils) to several weeks (e.g. erythrocytes) and several years (e.g. some lymphocytes). A balance between self-renewal and differentiation is important in order to avoid the emergence of cells that survive and grow in situations unfavourable for the growth of normal cells and hence to the establishment of diseases, for examples leukaemias (malignant proliferation of leukocytes).

Circulating and tissue cells of the immune system

As far as the immune system is concerned the two most important lineages are initiated from **lymphoid** and **myeloid** stem cells. A third lineage is of cells that show features belonging to both myeloid and lymphoid lines, one example of which are the natural killer (NK) cells.

• Many cells leaving the bone marrow possess little or no proliferative potential, that is, they cannot undergo further cell division.

• Erythrocytes and platelets do not contain genetic material (they have no nucleus) and neutrophils have condensed DNA and cannot undergo replication.

• Other haematopoietic cells, those of the lymphoid lineage, can undergo further replication and development in various tissues of the body.

Although pluripotential stem cells are still difficult to characterize morphologically, the cells ultimately produced by the bone marrow are most usually described by their appearance under a light microscope. They are very easily visualized using traditional Romanowsky stains. Cells of the myeloid lineage have the most diverse appearances (Figure 2.3a). When mature, they include the three types of **polymorphonuclear leukocyte (PMN)**, literally 'white cells with many-shaped nuclei', which are further subdivided according to their cytoplasmic granules into:

• neutrophils;
• eosinophils;
• basophils.

This nomenclature leads to the collective term **granulocyte** which is often used synonymously with PMN. All three granulocytic cell types exit from the bone marrow and enter the circulation as mature, competent cells. Unlike neutrophils and eosinophils, a further developmental stage is thought to exist for basophils which migrate from the circulation into tissues where they differentiate further to become **mast cells**. Mast cells (Figure 2.3b) are found in tissues throughout the body but they are fixed within tissues, not re-entering the circulation. The numbers of mast cells in tissues can be maintained either by further influx of basophils into tissues or by cell division *in situ*.

This characteristic of differentiating within tissues is also shared by the final cell type in the myeloid lineage: the **monocyte** (Figure 2.3c). This cell type is readily distinguishable from PMNs because it does not have either a segmented nucleus or cytoplasmic granules. When monocytes are stimulated to migrate into tissues they differentiate to become tissue **macrophages** (Figure 2.3d). Like

Consider the significance of the different nucleus:cytoplasm ratios of different leukocyte types. Cytoplasm is the part of the cell where macromolecules, especially proteins, are synthesized and prepared for secretion; where nutrients and other materials may be ingested into the cell and where a great deal of cellular metabolic activity takes place. The relative lack of cytoplasm in lymphocytes would indicate that protein secretion is not a significant function of these cells. Importantly, as we will see in Chapter 5, some lymphocytes can be stimulated to enter a phase where protein secretion is a vital role. Under such circumstances the cytoplasmic volume of the cell increases considerably.

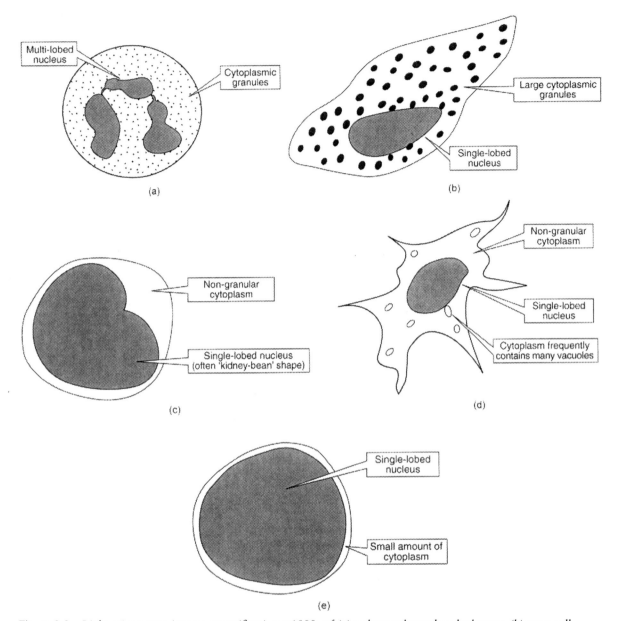

Figure 2.3 *Light microscopy images, magnification ×1000, of (a) polymorphonuclear leukocyte, (b) mast cell, (c) monocyte, (d) macrophage and (e) lymphocyte*

mast cells, macrophages do not re-enter the circulation. Macrophages are found in tissues throughout the body but their appearance and functions differ according to the tissue in which they occur. This phenomenon has led to a multiplicity of names for all of these so-called macrophage-like cells (Table 2.2). Together monocytes, macrophages and macrophage-like cells may be grouped under the collective term the **mononuclear phagocyte**

Table 2.2 *Macrophage-like cells*

Cell type	Location within the body
Kupffer cells	Liver
Histiocytes	Connective tissue
Glomerular mesangial cells	Kidney
Alveolar macrophages	Lungs
Osteoclasts	Bone
Splenic macrophages	Spleen
Synovial macrophages	Synovial joints
Langerhans cells	Skin (dermis)
Dendritic cells	Lymph nodes
Interdigitating cells	Lymph nodes

system. This term reflects both an important morphological feature of the cell types, i.e. a single nuclear shape, as well as an important function, phagocytosis (Chapter 3).

Lymphoid stem cells produce cells that differentiate to become **lymphocytes**. The morphological appearance of lymphocytes is distinct from other leukocytes in that they are approximately spherical and have only a very small amount of cytoplasm separating nuclear and plasma membranes (Figure 2.3e). Lymphocytes do not contain cytoplasmic granules. There are two different types of lymphocytes: **T lymphocytes** and **B lymphocytes**. These are commonly referred to as **T cells and B cells**. It not possible to distinguish T cells from B cells using light microscopy and conventional stains alone.

Not all of the maturation stages of lymphocytes occur within the bone marrow. T cells exit the bone marrow and circulate to the **thymus**, sometimes called the thymus gland where they are termed **thymocytes**. The entry-point to the thymus is in the **cortex** of each lobule of the organ (Figure 2.4). The thymus consists of two distinct lobes, each of which is subdivided into many lobules. Thymocytes then circulate through the thymus on a well-defined pathway during which they interact with many different cell types including thymic epithelial cells. During this circulation thymocyte maturation and differentiation take place. A detailed description and examination of the nature and purpose of thymic maturation is considered in Chapter 4. Mature T cells exit the thymus at the **medulla** and enter the circulation. In common with the other primary lymphoid tissue, the bone marrow, the thymus also degenerates during childhood. Its size and function are greatest in the young child but, by about the time of puberty, it is present only as a microscopic remnant.

The origins of the names 'T cells' and 'B cells' are interesting. T cells are so-called because, when they leave the bone marrow, they travel to another primary lymphoid organ, the thymus, to undergo further maturation. The 'T' then stands for thymus. For B cells the story is not so clear-cut. In 1956 the journal Poultry Science carried a brief, two-page article that linked the immune response of chickens with a small gut-associated organ known as the Bursa of Fabricius. Birds are the only creatures to possess this organ. Experiments carried out indicated that chickens whose Bursa had been removed showed immune deficiencies. Later it was shown that a class of lymphocytes matured in the Bursa. This was a very important finding as it indicated, for the first time, that lymphocytes were involved in immune responses. These became known as B lymphocytes. Humans do not have a Bursa so, for many years, a hot topic of research was to find the human 'Bursal-equivalent'. It is now widely considered that B cell maturation is completed in the bone marrow, happily giving us another 'B' word. Confoundingly, the mass of new information now emerging on the immune system of the human gut is re-awakening the possibility of a form of gut-associated lymphoid tissue which may contribute to lymphocyte maturation.

Figure 2.4 *One of the many lobules of the thymus. Immature T cells (thymocytes) enter via the bloodstream at the cortex and move through the lobule to exit into the peripheral circulation at the medulla. Interactions with the various cell types along this pathway induce thymocyte maturation*

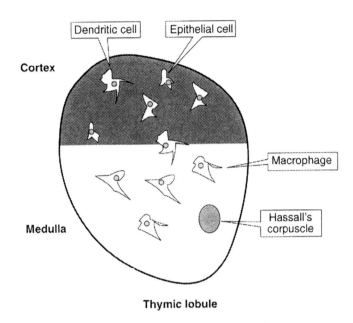

Thymic lobule

Relationships between lymphoid tissues and immune cells

The special roles of bone marrow and thymus in producing and maturing lymphocytes have led them to be called the **primary lymphoid tissues**. The other lymphoid tissues, **secondary lymphoid tissues** (Table 2.3) throughout the body are sites where mature lymphocytes congregate in close proximity with macrophage-like cells and other blood cell types. It is here that many immune responses take place. There is a real advantage in the positioning of the secondary lymphoid tissues at sites where contact with non-self material is likely to take place, for example lining the digestive tract, the respiratory tract and the genito–urinary tracts. These are the interfaces with the body's internal environment where each of the organs has a lining of mucosal tissue. The lymphoid tissue is collectively termed **mucosa-associated lymphoid tissue (MALT)**. Specialized MALT occurs along the digestive tract as **gut-associated**

Table 2.3 *Secondary lymphoid tissues*

Tonsils
Adenoids } Waldeyer's ring
Associated lymph nodes
Spleen (white pulp)
Gut-associated lymphoid tissues (GALT) including Peyer's patches
Mesenteric lymph nodes
Appendix
Other mucosa-associated lymphoid tissue (MALT)
Other lymph nodes

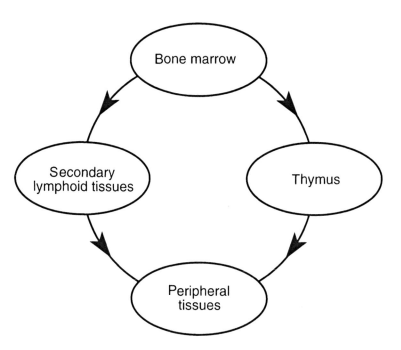

Figure 2.5 *Unlike other leukocyte types, lymphocytes can recirculate between the lymphoid tissues and other tissues of the body, although only T cells enter the thymus. Arrows indicate cell movement via the lymphatic vessels and blood vessels*

lymphoid tissue (GALT). The **spleen** is not associated with an external–internal interface, however it is highly rich in blood vessels (the red pulp). The spleen is where senescent (old and imperfect) erythrocytes are destroyed by the mononuclear phagocytes. The haemoglobin from the destroyed cells begins the conversion necessary for eventual excretion as pigments such as bilirubin. Thus the spleen is a filtration system. The white pulp, the lymphoid tissue, is found surrounding the blood vessels scattered throughout the whole organ. Thus the immune cells are ideally positioned to mount responses against any non-self that may be filtered from the blood stream.

Both T and B cells participate in a constant process of recirculation through vessels (lymphatic and cardiovascular) and tissues (secondary, lymphoid and peripheral) (Figure 2.5). Conversely, none of the other leukocyte types can re-enter the circulation once they have moved into peripheral tissues.

One type of secondary lymphoid tissue that is distributed throughout the body is found in lymph nodes. A lymph node (Figure 2.6) is a kidney-shaped structure that filters the lymph which passes through it. Lymph enters a node via afferent lymphatics and exits through efferent lymphatics, the number of afferent lymphatics always exceeding the number of efferent. Within the lymph node the **germinal centres** are well-organized foci of cells. As can be seen in Figure 2.6, the two types of lymphocyte accumulate preferentially in different areas of the node, T cells in the medulla and B cells in the cortex. During an immune response the number of leukocytes within a lymph node

Although the spleen performs very important functions, it is not essential for life. Located in the abdomen, it is the most easily injured of all the vital organs in that region. When the spleen is injured, as frequently occurs in traumatic accidents such as motorcycle crashes, it is so rich in blood vessels that the patient risks bleeding to death. Surgical removal of the spleen (splenectomy) usually prevents such deaths. Following splenectomy the rest of the immune system can take over the spleen's tasks. However, patients may have a subsequently raised chance of infection. In some hospitals patients who have undergone splenectomy may receive additional immunizations to minimize the risk of infection, however that is not current practice within the UK.

Figure 2.6 *Generalized structure of a lymph node showing the distinct locations of B cells and T cells. Lymph enters the node through afferent lymphatics and particulate matter, including cells, is filtered out. The resulting fluid exits through the efferent lymphatics*

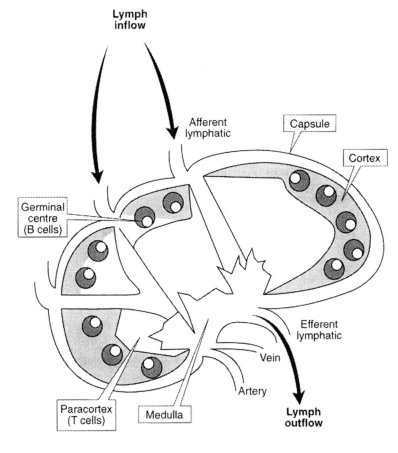

increases considerably. This is due both to the proliferation of lymphocytes within the germinal centres and through the arrival of new cells from the circulation. The ability of lymphocytes to proliferate in germinal centres greatly improves the speed and the intensity of a response. The evolution of germinal centres is considered to have been a very significant step. Mammals are the only animal species in which they are found and the mammalian immune response is considerably more effective than that of other species.

The filtration activity of the node allows the retention of any particulate material which has been transported from the tissues in the lymph. Particulate matter would include both self material (e.g. dead cells dislodged from tissues) and non-self material (e.g. bacterial cells). Tumour (cancer) cells may also be present. This entrapment of tumour cells in the lymph node is the reason why secondary cancer growths, known as **metastases**, are frequently found in the nodes. At surgery for removal of tumours the healthcare team always takes a biopsy sample of adjacent lymph nodes to ensure that they do not contain any metastatic growths. The tumour tissue and node samples would be sent to the

The movement of fluid and cells within the lymphatics and the release of leukocytes from lymph nodes was formerly considered to be passive, solely dependent on the contraction of adjacent muscles to squeeze the lymph along or the formation of new tissue fluid to exert a forward pressure. Now, however, it is recognized that the smooth muscle of lymphatics and lymph nodes is enervated. The role of the nervous system in stimulating the activities of the lymphatic system is an area of interesting research potential.

laboratory to undergo rapid examination for the presence of malignant cells. The test results would be transmitted immediately to the operating theatre so that if metastases are present, the affected lymph nodes can be excised together with the main tumour tissue. One very important skill of a pathologist or histopathologist is to be able to distinguish between a lymph node which is enlarged through the accumulation of cells during an ongoing immune response, known as a reactive lymph node, and one that is enlarged because it contains cancer cells. Cancers of blood cells, leukaemias and lymphomas, pose particular difficulties because the cells that are increased in number will resemble leukocytes proliferating during an immune response.

Non-cellular components of the immune system

Immune responses occur in virtually all parts of the body. We have seen that immunocompetent cells can travel throughout the body borne in the cardiovascular and lymphatic circulations. However, it is not always cells that are directly responsible for carrying out functions or for communicating with other cells during a response. There are several types of non-cellular factors, predominantly proteins, that also play very significant effector and regulatory roles.

One very large group of proteins that is important for immune and inflammatory responses is the **acute phase proteins (APP)**, sometimes also called acute phase reactants (APR). The term 'acute phase' derives from the fact that these proteins exert their effects usually during the acute, or early, part of responses. They are synthesized predominantly in the liver but also in macrophages. The APP may be sub-divided into a number of distinguishable groups, as shown in Table 2.4. We know the precise role within the immune response of many of the groups, for example, **complement** proteins (see Chapter 3). However, some other groups are even now identified only on the basis of their greatly increased concentrations during responses, for example, major APP. Nonetheless, the therapeutic monitoring of APP concentrations may assist in patient management. For example, a patient who undergoes severe trauma such as massive injury in a car crash will show extremely elevated

> What is complement? Complement is a series of more than 20 plasma proteins. The concentrations of complement rise during the acute phase of an immune or inflammatory response. The predominant protein is known as C3 and its concentration is normally greater than 1 mg per millilitre of plasma. Complement proteins are responsible for the destruction of non-self cells, especially bacteria. Complement can also help to regulate the responses of cells such as neutrophils, monocytes and macrophages.

Table 2.4 *Acute phase proteins (APPs)*

Complement proteins
Negative APP (suppress responses)
Haemostatic proteins (blood clotting)
Major APP (e.g. CRP, SAA)
Protease inhibitors
Metal-binding proteins
Other proteins (e.g. lipoprotein a, α_1 acid glycoprotein)

levels (up to a 1000-fold rise) of **C-reactive protein (CRP)**. By monitoring plasma levels of CRP the healthcare team can look for a return to normal values and so establish that the patient is recovering. Conversely, an unexpected resurgence of CRP levels may signal that the patient has contracted an infection and so can be treated rapidly. **Serum amyloid A (SAA)** is another major APP that is readily detected in plasma.

Cytokines

Cytokines are polypeptides and glycoproteins, usually of low molecular weight (less than 30 kDa), that are secreted from a range of cell types within the body. Membrane-bound forms have been described for many cytokines, and some may also be associated with the extracellular matrix. Cytokines act as messengers between those cells that secrete them and cellular targets. The number of known cytokines is still increasing and currently exceeds 50. Table 2.5 lists the principal cytokine families that have been characterized to date. It is important to remember that the production and function of cytokines are not confined to the immune system.

Table 2.5 *Cytokines*

Principal cytokine families	Family members	Cell source
Colony-stimulating factors	GM-CSF	T cells, macrophages, fibroblasts, mast cells, endothelial cells
	G-CSF	Fibroblasts, endothelial cells
	M-CSF	Fibroblasts, endothelial cells
Interferons	IFN-α	Leukocytes
	IFN-β	Fibroblasts
	IFN-γ	T cells
Interleukins	IL-1	Macrophages, fibroblasts
	IL-2	T cells
	IL-3	T cells, mast cells
	IL-4	T cells, mast cells, bone marrow
	IL-5	T cells, mast cells
	IL-6	T cells, macrophages, mast cells, fibroblasts
	IL-7	Bone marrow
	IL-8*	Monocytes
	IL-9	T cells
	IL-10	T cells, B cells, macrophages
	IL-11	Bone marrow
	IL-12	T cells
	IL-13	T cells
Transforming growth factors	TGF-α	T cells, B cells
	TGF-β	T cells, B cells
Tumour necrosis factors	TNF-α	Macrophages, T cells
	TNF-β	T cells

*IL-8 is also a member of the cytokine-like family known as chemokines.

Some of the functions of cytokines are the positive or negative regulation of cell proliferation, differentiation and, indeed, the regulation of immune responses. Many cytokines do not appear to have just a single function, these are said to be **pleiotropic**. Many of the sources and targets of cytokines are within the immune system, however cytokines may allow effective communication between the immune system and all of the other organ systems within the body. In fact, frequent reference is made to cytokines as the hormones of the immune system. This analogy with endocrine hormones, which travel in the bloodstream to a target organ where they exert an effect, has only limited usefulness when trying to understand the modes of action of cytokines. Under certain circumstances some cytokines behave like classical hormones in that they can act at a systemic level. In general, though, cytokines act on a wider spectrum of target cells than hormones and, unlike hormones, cytokines are not produced by cells that are organized in specialized glands, i.e. there is not a single organ source for each cytokine.

Cytokines *in vivo* function at nano- (10^{-9} M), pico- (10^{-12} M) or even femtomolar (10^{-15} M) concentrations (Chapter 3). It is important to note that excessively raised concentrations of cytokines can have severe damaging effects on the body and may even lead to death. One situation where high levels of cytokines enter the circulation with potentially lethal consequences is **septic shock** (septicaemia). The effects of cytokines upon their target cells depend upon cytokine receptors that are anchored within cellular cytoplasmic membranes. When the receptor is occupied by the appropriate cytokine ligand the cell's response is initiated. Cytokine antagonists have also been identified and these also play significant roles in the regulation of immune cell function. The short *in vivo* half-life of cytokines is thought to be due, in part, to the release of natural antagonists.

Suggested further reading

Gordon, S. (1995) The macrophage. *Bioessays* **17**, 977–986.

Griebel, P.J. and Hein, W.R. (1996) Expanding the role of Peyer's patches in B-cell ontogeny. *Immunology Today* **17**, 30–39.

Hall, S.S. (1997) A Commotion in the Blood. New York: Henry Holt.

Perry, M. and Whyte, A. (1998) Immunology of the tonsils. *Immunology Today* **19**, 414–421.

Peters, J.H., Gieseler, R., Thiele, B. and Steinbach, F. (1996) Dendritic cells: from ontogenic orphans to myelomonocytic descendants. *Immunology Today* **17**, 273–278.

Solomon, E.P. and Davis, W.P. (1983) Human Anatomy and Physiology. Holt-Saunders International edition (New York: CBS College Publishing), pp. 503–520.

How were cytokines discovered originally? In the 1970s, using the cell culture and biochemistry techniques that were then available, scientists observed that particular cells (target cells) *in vitro* could be stimulated to differentiate, to proliferate or to carry out specific functions. In order to stimulate these events the scientists used fluid in which other cells had grown previously, however the same fluid, unused for cell culture, could not act in the same way. These findings indicated that the stimulus for the observed events was biological molecule(s) produced by the original cells. Soluble biochemical species (protein) could be isolated from the cell culture that were deemed to be responsible for stimulating the target cells. The isolated proteins were often given names that related to their supposed effects, e.g. growth factors or differentiation factors. More recently, when proteins could be purified fully or synthesized in pure forms through molecular biology techniques, it was realized that each particular protein (now known as a cytokine) could exert many different effects (**pleiotropy**) and, complicating the picture still further, many different cytokines could have the same effect (**degeneracy**). A more rational system of nomenclature is now used for most cytokines (Table 2.5).

Self-assessment questions

1. List two important differences between the lymphatic system of a new-born child and that of an adult.
2. Describe the relationship between the lymphatic system and the cardiovascular system.
3. Distinguish between the polymorphonuclear leukocytes and the mononuclear phagocytes.
4. What are the most abundant leukocyte types within the circulating blood and what is the normal range of their count?
5. Discuss the relevance of the location of secondary lymphoid tissues within the body.
6. What are the origins of the names of the two classes of lymphocytes?
7. What is the principal site of acute phase protein (APP) synthesis and why are the major APP so-called? Give two examples of major APP.
8. How do cytokines mediate their effects on target cells?
9. Name two factors that may determine the effectiveness of a cytokine.
10. How were cytokines discovered?

Key Concepts and Facts

The Immune System
- The lymphatic system includes tissues, organs, connecting vessels and circulating cells that are important for mounting immune responses.

- Lymphoid tissues are the tissues of the lymphatic systems and the interconnecting vessels are the lymphatics.

Development of the Immune System
- In the foetus immune cells are produced in the liver.

- After birth the bone marrow is the site of haematopoiesis.

Production of Immune System Cells
- Pluripotential stem cells give rise to all blood cell types.

- Erythroid stem cells produce red blood cells.

- Myeloid stem cells produce polymorphonuclear leukocytes (PMN; granulocytes), monocytes and megakaryocytes (leading to platelets).

- Lymphoid stem cells produce B and T lymphocytes with the T cells undergoing maturation in the thymus.

- In the tissues monocytes differentiate into macrophages while basophils are thought to differentiate into mast cells.

Lymphoid Tissues
- Immune cells arise in the primary lymphoid tissues.

- Mature immune cells are located in organized regions within secondary lymphoid tissues and this is where most immune responses occur.

Non-cellular Components of the Immune System
- Synthesis of the acute phase proteins is increased during immune responses.

- Cytokines carry out many important immunological functions including communication between cells and tissues.

Chapter 3
Natural immune responses

Learning objectives

After studying this chapter you should confidently be able to:

Describe the primary signs and symptoms of acute inflammation.

Explain how the functions of cells and molecules lead to the observable signs and symptoms.

Explain how the immune system can kill through phagocytosis and complement activity.

Discuss how tissues and organs throughout the body may be involved in inflammation.

Understand that, in successful responses, tissues return to their normal state.

Describe the role of natural killer (NK) cells.

Acute inflammation

When foreign, or **non-self**, material is present in host, or **self**, tissues swift action must be taken to eliminate it. This action, **a response**, will greatly reduce any potential threat. The response will be terminated when all tissues are restored to the condition they were in prior to the contact with the non-self. It is critical that the first wave of responses should be concerned with speed and efficacy; the short-term threat must be removed regardless of the long-term consequences of that action. Obviously, if the long-term consequences were overwhelmingly damaging to the host, evolutionary pressures would likely have produced an inflammatory response which had built-in brakes and safeguards to limit the harm to the individual host. These brakes and safeguards do in fact exist within the human immune system. It can be said that we truly have a system which aims to inflict the maximum damage on the foreign 'invader' while minimizing damage to the self. This highly effective, but very well controlled, response is known as a natural immune response or, more commonly, **acute inflammation**.

Acute inflammation is a protective mechanism. This statement may be a bit difficult to accept in today's world in which the symptoms of inflammation are regarded as such a nuisance. Anti-inflammatory drugs, e.g. aspirin, comprise the single largest class of drugs consumed. The characteristic primary signs and symptoms of inflammation were recognized many years ago in ancient Rome when Cornelius Celsus described rubor, calor, dolor and tumour as the 'cardinal signs of inflammation'. These may be translated into medical terms of 'oedema, erythema, noxia and fever' and into everyday English as:

- swelling
- redness
- pain
- heat.

Rudolf Virchow, in the nineteenth century, added *function laesa* (**loss of function**) as the fifth cardinal sign of inflammation.

Initiation of inflammatory responses

In order to initiate a response against any foreign material that has entered the body, the cells of the immune system must be made aware of its presence. This signalling occurs through the release of small molecular weight chemicals termed **inflammatory mediators**. One source of these mediators is cells that have been damaged in the events which led to the introduction of the foreign body. Tissue cells, especially **mast cells**, are also rich sources of inflammatory mediators and others are derived from extracellular proteins, for example a protein fragment called C5a. This is an active enzyme released on hydrolytic breakdown of factor C5, a component of the **complement** series of proteins. There is constant, low-level break-down of C5 within extracellular fluids but the release of C5a from its inactive precursor is greatly increased during an immediate inflammatory response. The foreign bodies themselves, bacteria, for example, may release the potent inflammatory mediator **FMLP**. This is a sequence of the amino acids formylmethionine, leucine and phenylalanine that is produced when bacterial protein synthesis occurs. The presence of FMLP in any human tissue indicates that active bacterial metabolism is taking place.

Prostaglandins and other eicosanoids

Inflammation is often associated with disruption of the cell membrane phospholipids particular to a tissue. Membrane phospholipids are attacked by phospholipases to liberate arachidonate, the anion of arachidonic acid. Metabolism via different enzymes stimulates the arachidonic acid cascade which produces a group of molecules known as the **eicosanoids** (Figure 3.1). These are highly active but short-lived mediators of inflammation. They cannot be stored so they are not pre-formed. Inflammatory cells such as

> Mast cells are simulated to degranulate (release their granules) as a result of interactions of their cell membranes with extracellular molecules or other cells. The released granules then rupture releasing highly reactive small molecular weight molecules including histamine, heparin and serotonin as well as several enzymes.

> Eicosanoid synthesis is inhibited by non-steroidal anti-inflammatory drugs (NSAIDs) such as aspirin or ibuprofen, and by negative feedback loops. In contrast, positive feedback loops exist that allow for increased synthesis of the eicosanoids. Eicosanoids act close to the cells in which they are created and disappear quickly due to their rapid inactivation. The half-life of eicosanoids is generally less than five minutes. This allows the body to decrease or increase the amount of eicosanoids very quickly and to cause significant effects within a short time.

Figure 3.1 *The arachidonic acid cascade*

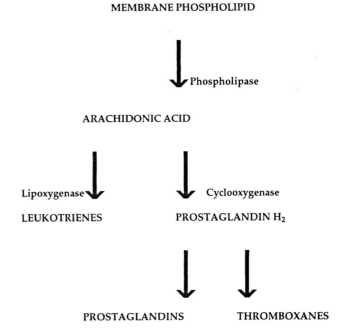

MEMBRANE PHOSPHOLIPID

Phospholipase

ARACHIDONIC ACID

Lipoxygenase   Cyclooxygenase

LEUKOTRIENES   PROSTAGLANDIN H_2

PROSTAGLANDINS   THROMBOXANES

monocytes are able to activate the arachidonate cascade to produce eicosanoids. This happens when monocytes move into a tissue and interact with the tissue's cells. Eicosanoids have a wide variety of functions. The cell type in which they are synthesized is an important regulator of eicosanoid production because the cell type defines the ratios and amounts of different enzymes that are active within the cell. Different enzymes lead to different eicosanoid products and, therefore, to different physiological processes.

There are three major types of eicosanoids:

- leukotrienes
- thromboxanes
- prostaglandins.

The **leukotrienes**, most commonly found in the leukocytes, mast cells, platelets and vascular tissue of the lung and heart, are produced by basophils and mast cells by breakdown of certain membrane phospholipids. Leukotrienes are involved in several inflammatory reactions and are constituents of substances originally called 'slow-reacting substance of anaphylaxis' (SRS-A). They contract smooth muscle, affect vascular permeability and are strong chemoattractants for neutrophils. Leukotrienes are more potent than histamine in constricting airways and promoting tissue oedema formation.

Thromboxanes constrict blood vessels, suppress cyclic AMP and promote platelet aggregation.

The **prostaglandins** (PGs) have many very specific roles in various tissue types. Prostaglandins of the E series are known to:

- dilate arterioles and capillaries to bring about a drop in blood pressure;
- relax vascular smooth muscle;
- open the bronchi of the lungs;
- enhance blood flow through the kidneys;
- increase urinary volume as well as the excretion of sodium ions;
- cause contraction of gut muscle.

The PGF series is known to:

- constrict venules which increases blood pressure;
- constrict the bronchi of the lungs;
- produce contractions of the uterus and induce abortion or labour at term.

The different prostaglandins exert their apparently contradictory effects by acting on different cellular mechanisms and not by antagonizing each other on the same mechanism.

The inhibition of eicosanoid synthesis is performed by **non-steroidal anti-inflammatory drugs (NSAIDs)** such as aspirin or ibuprofen, and by negative feedback loops. In contrast, positive feedback loops exist that allow for increased synthesis of the eicosanoids.

Molecules and cells interact

So, concurrent with cellular events, the inflammatory mediators also increase the diameter of blood vessels over a small area of tissue to promote blood flow to that area. This is **vasodilation**. The consequences to the individual of massive dilation may be significant, leading to shock, loss of consciousness or death. This is one reason why vasodilation usually occurs in post-capillary venules, rather than in capillaries: if capillaries were dilated the increased blood flow into the very large number of vessels in any one area, and away from vital organs such as the heart, lungs and brain, would lead rapidly to adverse consequences including fainting, coma and, if prolonged, death.

The small size of the inflammatory mediators allows them to diffuse through the tissues and away from the site of their release. Thus a chemical concentration gradient is established in which the highest concentration is at the point of release and the concentration decreases in proportion to the distance from that point. **Endothelial cells** that line the blood vessels respond rapidly to the presence of inflammatory mediators. The nature of the response is threefold (Figure 3.2):

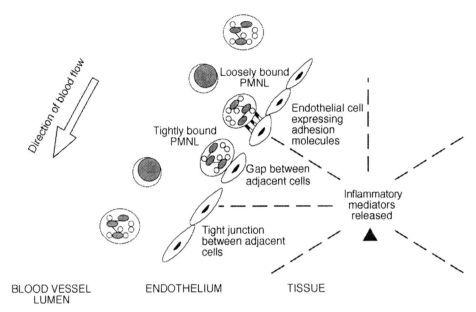

Figure 3.2 *Responses of endothelial cells to inflammatory mediators. PMNL, Polymorphonuclear leukocyte*

- endothelial cells change shape, becoming more rounded so that gaps appear between adjacent cells;
- endothelial cells begin to express adhesion molecules which make their inner (luminal) surfaces 'sticky';
- endothelial cells express soluble molecules, cytokines, that increase the rate and extent of the inflammatory response.

Adhesion molecules

The changes that take place in endothelial cells lead to one important phenomenon: they permit leukocytes from the blood stream to enter the tissues. Extensive endothelial cell–leukocyte interaction is necessary for this and **adhesion molecules** facilitate it. Over the past decade there has been immense progress in our understanding of adhesion molecules and their functions.

The adhesion molecules on the cell surface may be grouped into four major families. The **integrins** are membrane glycoproteins with two subunits, designated α (alpha) and β (beta). An important feature of integrins is that they exist in active and inactive states. An activated cell can transmit a signal from its cytoplasm that modifies the conformation of the extracellular domains of integrins on the cell membrane, increasing the affinity of the integrins for their ligands. This 'inside out' signalling occurs, for example, when leukocytes are stimulated by bacterial peptides, and it rapidly increases the affinity of the leukocyte integrins for molecules expressed on the leukocyte surface. Once the integrin has bound

Cells within tissues or in the circulation must interact with each other. This interaction is permitted by cell surface adhesion molecules. The expression and regulation of adhesion molecules controls many aspects of cell–cell communication and such important events as 'homing', i.e. the ability of a cell to move through the circulation and exit to a particular tissue. In general, contact through adhesion molecules results in the transmission of information that allows the cell to interact with its environment. Many microbial pathogens use adhesion

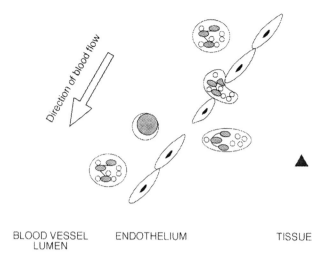

Figure 3.3 *Leukocytes are recruited from the circulation through interaction with endothelial cells and move through the tissue by chemotaxis*

BLOOD VESSEL   ENDOTHELIUM   TISSUE
    LUMEN

to its ligand 'outside in' signalling follows and affects many processes inside the cell, e.g. rearrangement of the cytoskeleton.

Members of the **immunoglobulin gene superfamily** contain highly conserved and easily recognizable peptide regions that are said to be 'immunoglobulin-like'. This name derives from the immunoglobulin molecules that are associated with acquired immune responses (Chapter 5). The **cadherins** establish molecular links between adjacent cells. They form zipper-like structures at membrane junctions where a cell makes contact with other cells. Finally, unlike most adhesion molecules, which bind to other proteins, the **selectins** interact with carbohydrate ligands on leukocytes and endothelial cells.

The well-controlled, coordinated functions of endothelial cells, adhesion molecules and leukocytes allow specific leukocytes to be attracted from the circulation and directed into the tissues where the foreign body is present (Figure 3.3).

molecules to penetrate mammalian cells. In the common cold the rhinovirus infects nasal epithelial cells by 'docking with' intercellular adhesion molecule-1 (ICAM-1) as its receptor. The interaction between the virus and ICAM-1 has been resolved at the atomic level, raising the hope of finding ways of blocking rhinovirus infection. Inhibitors of adhesion interactions involved in other diseases, e.g. in thrombosis (blood clotting within vessels) are also being sought.

Movement of leukocytes to the site of inflammation

Once the leukocyte has been directed to pass through the endothelial layer and into the tissues, it still must be given help to reach the site where the foreign body is present. This process is known as **chemotaxis**, which may be defined as:

directional cell movement along a chemical gradient.

Above, we saw how a chemical gradient was generated by the release, and diffusion from the site, of inflammatory mediators. Leukocytes carry cell surface receptors which allow them to interact with inflammatory mediators that stimulate this chemotaxis, e.g. FMLP and C5a. These same inflammatory mediators have yet another role to play before the inflammatory response can

Figure 3.4 *Phagocytosis*

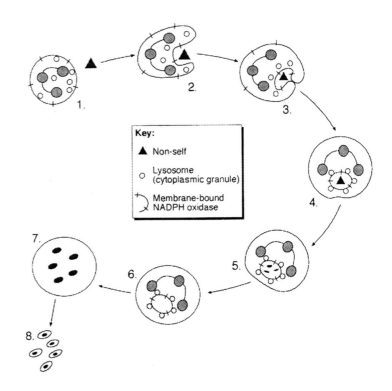

be considered to be exerting an effect. They must induce the activation of the leukocytes. The migration of cells is influenced by chemotactically active inflammatory mediators that are present in low concentrations. At higher concentrations, (10- to 100-fold), these mediators also induce a series of coordinated biochemical processes involving, for example, remodelling of the cytoskeleton and activation of enzymes. This is **cell activation**. It is important that it occurs only when the leukocyte has reached its target so as to avoid inappropriate interactions with host cells along its pathway through the tissue. Activation will lead, ultimately, to the elimination of the foreign body and one of the principal mechanisms by which this is achieved is phagocytosis. Characteristic signs of integrin signalling, i.e. protein phosphorylation, alteration of cytoplasmic pH and rearrangement of the cytoskeleton, herald the phagocytosis of a microorganism.

Phagocytosis

Elie Metchnikoff, in 1892, was the first to observe and study phagocytosis. The word 'phagocytosis' means, literally, cellular eating. What you will see is that this name could hardly be more apt involving, as it does, phases of ingestion, digestion and excretion. The overall process is depicted in Figure 3.4. The initial stage, ingestion, begins as a non-specific event with the interaction between leukocyte and target facilitated by diffusion events. Later, diffusion is replaced by more efficient, specific receptor-mediated interactions. This enhancement, termed **opsonization**, depends on some components of the complement system and antibodies from the acquired response (Chapter 5). At the end of the ingestion phase the foreign body is enclosed within a membranous sac, the **phagosome**, which was derived from the outer cell membrane of the leukocyte. The phagosome isolates the ingested foreign body in a separate compartment within the host cytoplasm. This important feature allows the next stage, digestion, to be directed solely towards the contents of the phagosome without the risk of altering any host cytoplasmic components.

Digestion involves the concerted action of an enzyme present on the phagosome membrane, **NADPH oxidase**, and the enzymes present in the cytoplasmic granules, or **lysosomes**. The lysosomes fuse with the phagosome membrane (Figure 3.4) to form a **phago-lysosome (or secondary lysosome)**, and their contents, predominantly **lysosomal enzymes**, are released into the space containing the ingested foreign material. Most of the lysosomal enzymes are acid hydrolases that are maintained in an inactive state through the high pH inside the lysosomes. In order for them to have an effect on the ingested materials, they must be activated. This requires the acidification of the phago-lysosomal contents and is facilitated by the products of the NADPH oxidase-catalysed reaction which is:

$$NADPH + O_2 \rightarrow NADP^+ + H^+ + O_2^-$$

Substrates for this reaction result from the increased leukocyte metabolism that is measurable when phagocytosis takes place and is characterized by:

- An increased (up to 20-fold) consumption of both O_2 and glucose.

- Increased activity of the metabolic pathway known as the **hexose monophosphate shunt (HMPS; pentose phosphate pathway)**, a major product of which is NADPH. One of the reaction products is $NADP^+$ and this re-enters the HMPS.

- Pumping of the H^+ across the phagosome membrane and into the phago-lysosome where it provides the decreased pH necessary for lysosomal acid hydrolase activation. The production of **reactive oxygen species (ROS)** one of which is O_2^-, or superoxide anion.

Together these events constitute the **respiratory burst**. Superoxide anion is the first one-electron reduction product of molecular oxygen. Further important ROS produced through subsequent reactions include H_2O_2 (**hydrogen peroxide**) which is also used as a general disinfectant on cuts and wounds in hospitals and at home. The ROS produced *in vivo* contribute to the elimination of ingested material by reacting with, and killing, any live microorganisms present in the phago-lysosome. In neutrophils, though not in any other phagocytes, another enzyme, **myeloperoxidase**, is present.

> NADPH oxidase is a complex enzyme. It consists of a number of membrane-bound and cytoplasmic components that are assembled on activation. It resembles the electron transport chain of oxidative phosphorylation that is found on the inner mitochondrial membrane.

> The organization of electrons in an oxygen molecule cause it to be highly reactive, participating in oxidation reactions where it itself is reduced. When the reduction involves only one electron, reactive oxygen species (ROS) are formed. Further oxidations–reductions may follow in one-electron steps. Each step causes the formation of ROS that are more highly reactive than in the previous step.

Figure 3.5 *Neutrophil apoptosis*

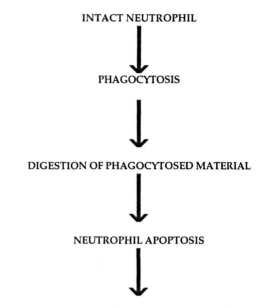

INTACT NEUTROPHIL

PHAGOCYTOSIS

DIGESTION OF PHAGOCYTOSED MATERIAL

NEUTROPHIL APOPTOSIS

INGESTION OF APOPTOTIC BODIES BY MONOCYTE / MACROPHAGES

Myeloperoxidase catalyses the interaction of ROS with halogens to form another series of toxic molecules, for example HOCl, hypochloric acid. The combined action of ROS and acid hydrolases ensures the compete digestion of the ingested materials. The resulting proteins, lipids, carbohydrates and nucleic acids are recycled for use within the phagocyte.

The final cellular stage in the acute inflammatory response is the removal of the infiltrating leukocytes (neutrophils) from the inflammatory site so that the host tissue may be restored to its original condition. This occurs by the process of **apoptosis**, a form of programmed cell death, in which the neutrophils orchestrate their own death in a genetically determined way (Figure 3.5). The end-result of apoptosis is the presence of **apoptotic bodies,** small membrane-bound packages of cytoplasm and nuclear material. These apoptotic bodies are rapidly removed from the tissue either by simple endocytosis into surrounding cells or by phagocytosis by infiltrating **macrophages.** One important feature of apoptotic bodies is that they do not act as inflammatory stimuli so that no new acute response is initiated.

Not all leukocytes infiltrate tissues simultaneously. Figure 3.6 shows a generalized time-course for the arrival at the inflammatory site of different types of leukocytes. Neutrophils are the first to accumulate followed by the mononuclear leukocytes, initially monocytes and macrophages then lymphocytes. Monocytes are phagocytic, but weakly so. Macrophages, when activated, are the most powerful phagocytes in the tissues. A significant difference between macrophages and neutrophils is that macrophages do not

Apoptosis is a form of programmed cell death, or cell suicide. Discovered over a quarter of a century ago, its true biological significance is only now appreciated. Apoptosis features in normal growth and development in many cells and tissues of both lower and higher animals. It occurs during embryo development and in the maturation of immune cells. Its regulation involves the products of many genes. In general, the genes belong to families of either death promoters or death inhibitors. Signals from a cell's environment may control the balance of activities between these two types of gene families.

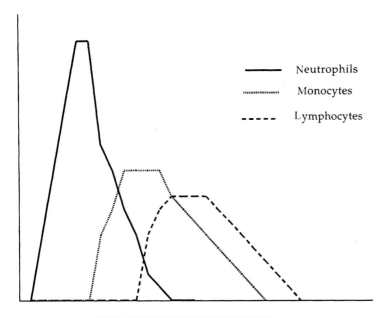

DURATION OF INFLAMMATION

Figure 3.6 *A generalized time course for the accumulation of different types of leukocytes at the inflammatory site*

undergo apoptosis following phagocytosis. When the acute inflammatory response comes to an end, it is likely that the macrophages continue their migration through the tissues. The cellular content of the inflammatory site is then restored to the state it was in prior to the arrival of the foreign material.

Cytokines in acute inflammation

With the initial release of inflammatory mediators, endothelial cells, leukocytes and fibroblasts respond by greatly increasing the synthesis and release of soluble messages, cytokines. Much of the responsibility for the overall integration of inflammatory responses lies with the **cytokines**. The principal pro-inflammatory cytokines are:

- interleukin-1 (IL-1)
- interleukin-6 (IL-6)
- interleukin-8 (IL-8)
- tumour necrosis factor α (TNF-α).

It is important to realize that cytokines tend to be related not so much by molecular or chemical structure but according to function. Cytokines may function in autocrine, intracrine, paracrine or juxtacrine manners (Figure 3.7). **Autocrine** is autostimulatory control in which a cell secretes a soluble factor that binds to its receptor, which is also expressed by the factor-producing cell. This creates a loop in which a cytokine acts back on the cells that

Figure 3.7 *Modes of action of cytokines*

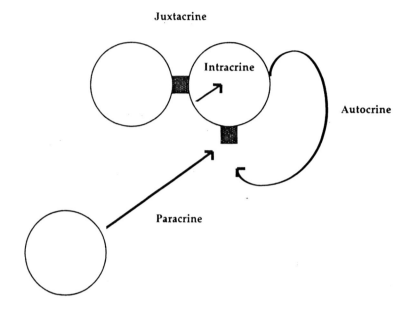

produced it. Interleukin-2 (IL-2), in acquired responses (Chapter 5) acts in this manner. **Intracrine** stimulation involves an internal autocrine loop requiring the presence of suitable intracellular biologically active receptors. The mechanisms underlying intracrine growth control are largely unknown but they might involve direct modulation of DNA replication and/or transcription. In **paracrine** stimulation the cytokine is secreted by a cell adjacent to the target cell. **Juxtacrine** regulation involves specific cell-to-cell contacts via a membrane-bound form of a cytokine that is normally secreted and a receptor on an adjacent cell. The membrane-bound cytokine then elicits the same spectrum of responses as the soluble cytokine. In fact, the membrane-bound form is frequently an incompletely processed, biologically active precursor of the secreted form of the factor. Examples of cytokines that may act in a juxtacrine manner are IL-1 and TNF-α. Juxtacrine interactions are probably also involved in the control of haematopoiesis (blood cell formation), allowing specific interactions between haematopoietic cells and the surrounding bone marrow stromal cells.

In vivo cytokines interact almost promiscuously with other cytokines and non-cytokines. There are additive, synergistic, co-operative, and antagonistic consequences of these interactions to yield what is commonly referred to as 'the cytokine network'. For example:

- IL-1 and interferon γ (IFN-γ, from acquired response) reduce some of the effects of IL-6.
- Some of the effects of IL-2 and IL-6 are antagonized by transforming growth factor β (TGF-β).

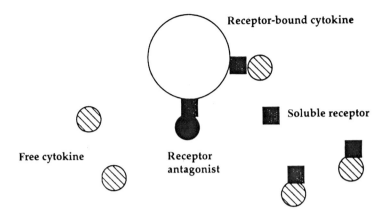

Figure 3.8 *Cytokine antagonists*

The combined action of two or even more cytokines may produce effects that no factor on its own would be able to achieve, although this is most readily demonstrated under *in vitro* conditions. For example:

- In cultured HepG2 hepatoma cells IL-1, IL-6, TNF-α and TGF-β induce the synthesis of the enzyme antichymotrypsin and at the same time inhibit the synthesis of albumin and alpha-foetoprotein (AFP).

- The synthesis of the blood clotting protein fibrinogen is induced by IL-6 and this effect is, in turn, suppressed by IL-1, TNF-α and TGF-β.

Once a cytokine interacts with its specific receptor on a cell surface, a signal is transmitted across the cytoplasmic membrane. Receptor-associated intracellular second messengers then translocate the signal to the nucleus leading to the activation of specific genes. The second messenger systems used following cytokine–receptor interactions are common to many cytokine and hormone receptors, e.g. the cyclic nucleotide or inositol phosphate pathways. It is currently unclear how the specificity of such signalling mechanisms is maintained. For many of the known cytokines the components of the signalling system have not been entirely characterized.

At least two types of **cytokine antagonist** are known (Figure 3.8): soluble cytokine receptors and cytokine receptor antagonists.

Soluble receptors are shed from the surface of cells and they interact with their cytokine ligand in solution. Thus the effective concentration of the cytokine is greatly reduced. One example of a soluble receptor system is the TNF receptor. There are two different types of TNF receptor, the 55 kDa receptor and the 75 kDa receptor. It is not yet clear why there are two receptor types, however both may be shed to act as TNF antagonists.

Receptor antagonists are molecules that bind to the receptor thus competitively inhibiting the cytokine ligand. The IL-1 receptor antagonist (IL-1RA) was the first of these to be reported. The *in vivo* concentration of IL-1RA may exceed that of IL-1.

Most cytokines have multiple target sites throughout the body on which their specific receptors are found. The principal targets of pro-inflammatory cytokines are the hepatocytes of the liver. One function of hepatocytes is to synthesize many types of protein. Hepatocytes respond to pro-inflammatory cytokines by upregulating their production of a diverse array of proteins, termed **acute phase proteins** (APP, Chapter 2). Each hepatocyte has the capacity to produce the entire spectrum of APP which are then secreted into the bloodstream. Following stimulation of single hepatocytes within individual hepatic lobules further hepatocytes are stimulated. This process continues until almost all hepatocytes produce APP and release them into the circulation.

The co-ordinated expression of many APP as a direct consequence of the activities of several cytokine stimuli can be explained, at least in part, by the fact that the regulatory sequences of the genes encoding APP contain so-called cytokine response elements. These response elements are recognized specifically by **transcription factors** that regulate the activity of these genes in a cell- and/or tissue-specific manner.

The general functions of APP are to:

- regulate immune responses;
- act as mediators and inhibitors of inflammatory processes;
- act as transport proteins for products generated during the inflammatory process;
- play an active role in wound tissue repair and tissue remodelling.

Complement is one component of human immune responses that is particularly effective in the rejection of mismatched tissue transplants. To overcome the shortage of human organs suitable for transplantation, attempts are being made to develop xenotransplants, i.e. the use of tissues from non-human sources. The pig is considered to be a possible source of tissues, however its use is restricted because human complement rapidly targets the porcine cells. A potential solution is to produce pigs that are genetically engineered to express human complement-degrading proteins on their cell surfaces.

Complement is a series of approximately 30 plasma proteins that are secreted as inactive APP. Their activation is by limited proteolytic cleavage and normally there is a slow but constant activation caused by the non-specific hydrolytic activities of many enzymes in plasma or extracellular fluids. During the acute inflammatory response, however, the rate of complement activation increases many-fold. Complement activation, or fixation as it is sometimes called, can proceed by three distinct pathways.

The **classical pathway** requires the presence of antibodies, which are products of acquired responses while the **alternate pathway** and **lectin pathway** are initiated during inflammatory responses on contact with, for example, bacterial cell surfaces. In evolutionary terms, the alternate pathway is probably the more ancient but the naming is an artefact of their sequence of discovery. The lectin pathway is the most recently described.

All pathways share a number of common important features. Figure 3.9 depicts complement activation by both classical and alternate pathways. It can be seen that factor C3 is pivotal in both pathways and is the most abundant of the complement proteins,

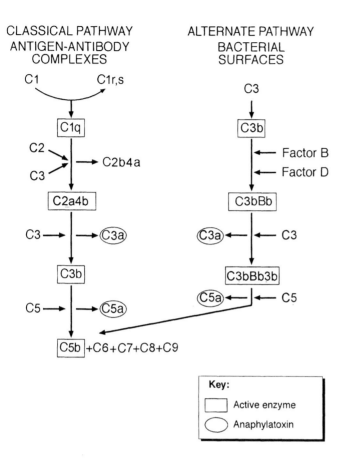

Figure 3.9   *Complement activation*

reaching concentrations of up to 1 mg per mL of blood plasma during the acute phase of a response.

The functions of complement are to:

- kill target cells;
- regulate inflammatory responses by enhancing phagocytosis and increasing leukocyte recruitment from the circulation.

Complement-mediated cell killing is achieved through formation of the final membrane attack complex (MAC) which is common to all activation pathways. The MAC forms a channel, or cylinder, with a hydrophilic core (Figure 3.10). When inserted into the lipid bi-layer of a target cell plasma membrane the normally continuous hydrophobic barrier is disrupted. The passage of charged particles between the interior and the exterior of the target cannot then be controlled. When many of these MAC are present on a single cell, the normal ionic gradients are disrupted and the cell dies.

Host cells take many precautions against the possibility of non-specific damage by complement. These precautions include:

Figure 3.10 *The membrane attack complex (MAC) of complement forms a channel, or cylinder, with hydrophilic core*

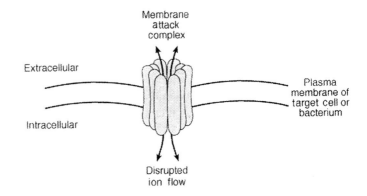

- The existence of complement inhibitors, especially C1 inhibitor (C1INH) that restricts the extent of activation via the classical pathway. This is a member of the serpin family (serine protease inhibitor) that also includes anti-thrombin III and α_1-antitrypsin. In the circulation most of the C1 is bound to C1INH so spontaneous initiation of the classical pathway is greatly reduced.

- The anchoring of complement proteins to the target cell surface by attachment to antibodies (classical pathway).

- The expression of cell surface proteins that interact with complement proteins to inactivate or degrade them. These factors are listed in Table 3.1 and are effective against both classical and alternate pathways of complement activation. They are called regulators of **complement activity (RCA)** and they reduce the activation of C3 and C5. Human RCAs are absent from the surfaces of, for example, bacteria. A bit confusingly, bacterial surfaces are said to be 'protected', the word 'protected' referring to the fact that the complement proteins are protected against degradation.

- Inhibition of the insertion of MAC into lipid bi-layer membranes. This is the function of molecules such as CD59 (interferes with C8–C9 interactions); vitronectin and SP-40,40.

Table 3.1 *Human cell surface regulators of complement activity*

Name	Activity
Decay accelerating factor (DAF)	Prevents formation of C3 convertase (classical + alternate)
C4 binding protein (C4bp)	Prevents formation of C3 convertase (classical). Degradation of C4b
Complement receptor 1 (CR1)	Prevents formation of C3 convertase (classical + alternate). Degradation of C3b and C4b
Factor H	Prevents formation of C3 convertase (alternate). C3b degradation
Membrane co-factor protein (MCP)	Degradation of C3b and C4b

Phagocytosis is enhanced when MAC and other complement proteins on cell surfaces act as **opsonins**. This is effective because neutrophils and macrophages express receptors for complement, principally **C3b receptors**, so bind readily to cells with C3b on the surface.

The recruitment of leukocytes from the circulation is enhanced by the small fragments cleaved from factors C2, C3 and C5. These are potent inflammatory mediators and also cause vasodilation (increased diameter of blood vessels so that blood flow to a region is increased). Fragments **C2a, C3a and C5a** are called **anaphylatoxins** and the most potent is C5a. At the site where inflammatory mediators interacted with endothelial cells, the increased blood flow and the gaps between adjacent lining cells permit the fluid phase of blood (plasma) to pass into the tissues. This is known as the **inflammatory exudate**. The exudate is rich in proteins: normal plasma proteins, the APP released from the liver and cytokines. This system for the delivery of proteins to the inflammatory site is extremely important for the successful progress of the response.

Once complement activation gets underway and MAC are formed, it is essential that the activation is down-regulated so that excessive cell killing or inflammation is not promoted. The down-regulation occurs through:

- specific inhibitors of complement activation;
- proteolytic cleavage to degrade already-formed active fragments.

Cleaved fragments of complement components also have regulatory functions within inflammatory responses. These functions are expressed because of the occurrence of specific complement receptors on the surfaces of leukocytes and other cell types, for example, endothelial cells.

Chemokines are multipotent cytokines that localize and enhance inflammation. They induce chemotaxis and activation of different types of inflammatory cells typically present at inflammatory sites. Chemokines also are secreted by these inflammatory cells. Chemokines may prime immune cells to respond to sub-optimal amounts of other inflammatory mediators while also stimulating inflammatory mediator release from leukocytes.

> Chemokines exert their effects on distinct subsets of cells. C–X–C chemokines, for example, appear to attract neutrophils but not macrophages, while C–C chemokines preferentially induce migration of macrophages. It is now assumed that the combined effects of multiple chemokines and other mediators are responsible for the cellular composition at inflammatory sites.

Wound healing

Inflammation is said to have ended successfully, or resolved, when no structural cells have been lost and foreign materials have been removed. When the tissue has been damaged during the inflammatory process or in other ways, but the body itself is still alive, the tissue will either regenerate, i.e. wound healing, or be repaired by fibrous tissue.

If no fibrous tissue is required, the word 'resolution' is also appropriate. If any repair by fibrous tissue does occur, there will be a **scar**. Scar tissue is known by different names according to its site, e.g. cicatrix, fibrosis, adhesions, gliosis, fibroplasia. The principal components of the wound healing process are:

- migration of different cell types into the wound region;
- growth stimulation of epithelial cells and fibroblasts;
- formation of new blood vessels;
- generation of a new extracellular matrix.

The first step in wound healing is the activation of the blood clotting cascade, leading to **haemostasis** with a fibrin gel matrix (a clot) that can be colonized by inflammatory cells such as neutrophils, monocytes and macrophages. Thrombin inside the clot induces platelets to degranulate, i.e. to release the contents of their alpha-granules. These contain cytokines, e.g. **platelet-derived growth factor (PDGF)** which aid in tissue regrowth.

A brake is applied to the process of clot formation by a series of inhibitors such as **protein C**, **protein S** and **antithrombin III**. Dissolution of the clot is triggered by the production of plasmin, a powerful proteolytic enzyme which digests fibrin. Smooth muscle cells also contribute to terminating the clotting process by releasing prostaglandins which, in turn, prevent platelet aggregation and inhibit PDGF synthesis. Several chemotactic cytokines induce the migration of neutrophils and monocytes into the injured areas. The monocytes are differentiated into macrophages that secrete more cytokines including PDGF and **transforming growth factor β (TGF-β)**, which is a strong chemoattractant for monocytes and fibroblasts. Many macrophage-derived cytokines promote the further migration of inflammatory cells into the wound area. Transforming growth factor β also appears to be the major factor responsible for the formation of granulation (new) tissue and the synthesis of proteins of the extracellular matrix. The formation of new blood vessels within the wound area is stimulated for as long as required by various **angiogenesis** factors and epithelial tissue replacement is mediated by the **epidermal growth factor (EGF)** family of growth factors.

In the final phase of wound healing granulation tissue is gradually replaced by connective tissue, again under the influence of cytokines. The tissue has now been restored to the state it was in prior to its encounter with foreign material.

Natural killer cells

These cells that bear some resemblance both to lymphocytes and to monocytes, but are different to either, contribute to natural immune responses. They are sometimes called **large granular lymphocytes**. The natural killer (NK) cells kill tumour cells and normal virus-infected cells. Natural killer cells target any other cells

---

> All stages in wound healing depend critically on the biological activities of various cytokines, including chemokines, epidermal growth factor (EGF), fibroblast growth factor (FGF), platelet-derived growth factor (PDGF) and transforming growth factor (TGF). These cytokines function in a controlled manner to activate cells, act as chemoattractants, regulate cell growth and mediate signalling between immune cells and the nervous system.

that do not carry surface molecules, termed MHC Class I antigens (Chapter 4), that belong to the host. Many viruses switch off MHC Class I antigens and tumour cells typically do not have MHC Class I. Thus these are the two cell types that are attacked by NK cells. The killing of targets by NK involves the release of granules containing enzymes that break down the DNA of targets.

Suggested further reading

Gale, L.M. and McColl, S.R. (1999) Chemokines: extracellular messengers for all occasions? *Bioessays* **21**, 17–28.

MacMicking, J., Xie, Q-W. and Nathan, C. (1997) Nitric oxide and macrophage function. *Annual Review of Immunology* **15**, 323–350.

Sacks, G., Sargent, I. and Redman, C. (1999) An innate view of human pregnancy. *Immunology Today* **20**, 114–118.

Tilg, H., Dinarello, C.A. and Mier, J.W. (1997) IL-6 and APPs: anti-inflammatory and immunosuppressive mediators. *Immunology Today* **18**, 428–432.

Self-assessment questions

1. List the four primary signs of acute inflammation.
2. What is FMLP, what is its origin and what effect does it have when present in tissues?
3. What is the site of action of aspirin? To what group of drugs does it belong?
4. How do endothelial cells respond when stimulated by inflammatory mediators?
5. What is chemotaxis and what is its role in promoting acute inflammation?
6. What is opsonization? Name one opsonin that is a component of acute inflammation.
7. What enzyme is responsible for the respiratory burst of phagocytes? Discuss how the array of ROS produced in macrophages differs from that in neutrophils.
8. What is the principal target organ of pro-inflammatory cytokines?
9. Why is complement factor C3 so vital? What would be the likely consequences to an individual born with a profound C3 deficiency?
10. Give the correct sequence of stages in wound healing.

Key Concepts and Facts

Acute inflammation
- Acute inflammation is a protective response that involves the coordinated action of cells, soluble molecules and the vascular system.

- The protein synthetic activity of the liver is vital to the inflammatory response.

- The presence of non-self (foreign) material in tissues causes the release of inflammatory mediators.

- The response of endothelial cells to inflammatory mediators is critical to the initiation of the acute inflammatory response.

- Phagocytosis involves the ingestion, killing and digestion of foreign material.

- The respiratory burst of phagocytes is the enzyme-catalysed synthesis of reactive oxygen species (ROS) that can kill phagocytosed microorganisms.

- Pro-inflammatory cytokines, principally IL-1, IL-6 and TNF-α, are responsible for the overall coordination of inflammatory responses.

- Complement proteins are acute phase proteins that effectively kill target cells and enhance inflammatory responses.

- Host cells are resistant to the killing effects of complement.

- The movement of fluid from the vascular system is facilitated by gaps between endothelial cells. The fluid is the inflammatory exudate and it carries the soluble factors, e.g. cytokines and APP, that are essential for effective responses.

NK Cells
- NK cells target tumour cells and virus-infected cells.

Wound Healing
- Wound healing is the final stage in an acute inflammatory response. It restores a tissue to the state it was in prior to its infection with non-self.

Chapter 4
Immunological recognition

Learning objectives

After studying this chapter you should confidently be able to:

Provide an acceptable definition of the terms 'antigen' and 'epitope'.

Describe the general structure and function of the major groups of cell surface molecules involved in immune responses and the genes that encode these molecules.

Discuss the origins of diversity in the immune system

Describe how antigen is processed and presented in preparation for immune responses.

Understand the concept of immunological tolerance and discuss its origins.

Natural immune responses are highly effective at providing a first line of defence against non-self that may enter the body. The complete immune system is, however, considerably more complex and effective. This necessary complexity is the responsibility of the **acquired immune response**.

Before reaching an understanding of the functions and regulation of acquired responses it is necessary to know the many components and concepts that underlie this highly evolved system. This knowledge will also allow a clear picture to develop of how natural and acquired responses interact to provide a seamless, highly effective, defence and prevention system.

Understanding self and non-self

An initial, apparently simple, question might be 'What is it that humans are immune to?'. An equally simple answer, based upon an individual's personal experience could be 'Humans are immune to things that would cause disease or other harm'. For many years immunologists rejected the possibility of this simple answer and worked instead towards defining a model of the immune system that involved the **recognition** of what is 'self' and what is 'non-self',

In 1994 an American immunologist, Dr Polly Matzinger, and her colleagues, tried to develop a new concept of immunity that would not leave so many questions unanswered. This new model proposed that the immune system can recognize what is potentially harmful to the body and eliminate it. At the time of writing this 'danger' theory is the focus of intense debate and speculation worldwide amongst eminent immunologists. Many of those who would oppose the danger theory agree that the self/non-self hypothesis is incomplete: they just believe that there is no experimental evidence to support the danger theory. Matzinger and others are now devising new experiments that would test the theory and provide evidence either to support or reject it. Whether the theory is right or wrong, its proposal has spurred scientists to address some of the most fundamental questions in relation to how our bodies defend themselves.

with the consequent **destruction and elimination** of non-self. With this model it becomes necessary to define what is 'self' and what is 'non-self'. A generally acceptable definition of 'self' is:

everything that is in the body from about the time of birth. 'Non-self' would then be everything else in the universe, both known and unknown!

Unfortunately the shortcomings of the current 'self' definition become apparent when scrutinized by straightforward questions such as 'What about all the new things that appear in the body at puberty or pregnancy or when lactation begins?'. Are these self or non-self? If they are non-self, why are they not destroyed and eliminated by the body? Also, what about exogenous foodstuffs that are incorporated into the body? By definition, these are non-self yet we know they are only very rarely rejected. However, until a new radical insight is provided into the nature of acquired responses the working definitions given above are sufficient for consideration of most aspects of human immune responses.

In discussing the nature of acquired immune responses, it is necessary to grasp the currently acceptable definitions of a number of very important terms.

Antigen: This is an immunological term that may generate confusion for students, in part because of its conflicting use, not just in different texts, but often in different parts of a single text. The definition used throughout the current text is:

Antigen is anything that can be recognized by the immune system. Thus antigen can either be part of the host or can be foreign (i.e. self antigen or non-self antigen).

Epitope: The immune system does not recognize all parts of an antigen simultaneously. Rather recognition involves the interaction of specific parts of individual molecules on the surface of an immune cell with specific parts of molecules on an antigen. Each part of the antigen is regarded as being an **antigenic determinant**; so the antigen is composed of a series of antigenic determinants, or **epitopes**.

Epitope is the part of the antigen that is recognized by the immune system.

It will be evident that epitopes must be on the outer surface of the antigen. For example, if the antigen is a bacterial cell, the epitopes will be parts of molecules that compose the outer wall of the bacterium. The immune system recognizes some epitopes more easily than others; those most easily recognized are known as **immunodominant epitopes**. Several factors may contribute to the immunodominance of an epitope including:

- Its size. Larger epitopes are more likely to be recognized.
- Its density on the antigen surface. The more copies of the epitope that are present, the more immunodominant it is.

Cell surface molecules involved in the immune response

Many of the responses of the immune system involve interactions of cell surface molecules. The principal molecules to be considered belong to three groups:

- immunoglobulin (Ig), also known as the B cell receptor for antigen (BCR) on B cells;
- the T cell receptor for antigen (TCR) on T cells;
- Major Histocompatibility Complex (MHC) antigens on many cell types.

A system for naming cell surface molecules

Considering the vital importance to immune responses of cell surface molecules, it is not surprising that a clear system for naming those molecules has been developed.

The **CD** system is an organized classification which allows molecules to be named alphanumerically such that the same molecule, when present on different cell types, always has the same name. The letters 'CD' stand for 'cluster of differentiation', i.e. a macromolecule on a cell which has appeared during the process of differentiation of that cell.

All of the CD molecules participate, in some way, in immune responses. When a molecule is characterized, the scientist who has 'discovered' it is able to refer to the database of CD names and structures in order to determine whether or not it is a novel molecule. New molecules are verified and named by participants at periodic international CD workshops. This excellent system prevents the widespread confusion that would reign if every molecule was named individually by independent scientists. Table 4.1 lists just a small set of molecules defined by the CD system; the total number is now about 200.

The presence of each CD molecule may be detected using specific reagents based upon antibodies that bind to just a single CD molecule (monoclonal antibodies). It is important to remember that the CD group is the cell surface molecule, not the antibody. For example, in the case of molecule CD4 on T cells, an antibody which can bind to it may be termed 'anti-CD4 antibody'. The T cell which carries (expresses) the CD4 molecule is called a **CD4 positive** ($CD4^+$) **T cell**. The nature of a cell population may now be resolved by determining whether or not particular CD molecules are present on the cell surfaces.

The immunoglobulin gene superfamily

Figure 4.1 details the generalized structure of the cell surface molecules which belong to the **immunoglobulin gene superfamily**.

Table 4.1 *Some cell surface molecules as defined by the CD system*

Antigen	Occurs on
CD1	Thymocytes, dendritic cells
CD2	T cells, NK cells
CD3	T cells
CD4	Some T cells, macrophages, macrophage-like cells
CD8	Some T cells
CD11a	Leukocytes
CD11b	Granulocytes, monocytes, NK cells
CD11c	Granulocytes, monocytes, NK cells
CD19	B cells
CD21	B cells
CD22	B cells
CD25	Activated T cells, activated B cells, macrophages
CD65	Monocytes, macrophages
CD120a	55 kDa TNF receptor
CD120b	75 kDa TNF receptor

A gene superfamily is a group of genes encoding proteins that have structural and functional similarities.

It is thought that, way back in evolution, a primordial gene existed which underwent mutations, including duplications, to produce a family of related genes. Each of these was then subject to mutation and change. The genes which conferred advantages have been highly conserved and now occur on many cells that are involved in immunity. The basic structural similarities between all of these proteins are:

- an intracellular (cytoplasmic) hydrophilic anchor region;
- a membrane-spanning hydrophobic region;
- an extracellular hydrophilic region.

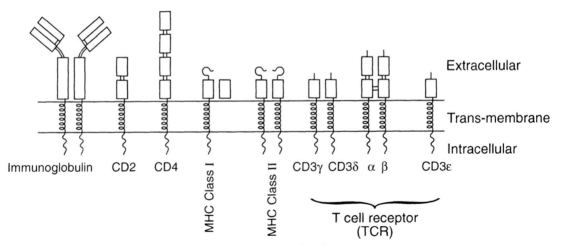

Figure 4.1 *Some members of the immunoglobulin gene superfamily*

The extracellular component is constructed from various combinations of a simple building block. The building block is termed an **immunoglobulin domain**. A domain is a peptide chain approximately 100 amino acids long, folded into a characteristic shape through intra-chain disulphide bridges. The shape of the Ig domains includes two layers of β-pleated sheet and three or four strands of antiparallel polypeptide chain.

The three classes of molecules that we are now considering, i.e. TCR, Ig and MHC, all belong to this group.

Immunoglobulin

Immunoglobulin (Ig) is a globular protein, commonly referred to as **antibody**. Its *in vivo* conformation is complex. Figure 4.2 shows a simple schematic structure of an Ig molecule. It comprises four peptide chains; two of lesser molecular weight (light chains) and two heavier (heavy) chains. The molecule has well-defined regions. Elucidation of the biochemical structure of immunoglobulins and the first description of the relationship between structure and function came in the late 1950s. Sir Rodney Porter, who was awarded the 1972 Nobel Prize for Medicine, developed a technique whereby Ig molecules could be cleaved enzymatically into distinct fragments, each of which retained biological activity (Figure 4.3). This approach, combined with that of Edelman in the United States, who used a different proteolytic enzyme (pepsin) to cleave the Ig molecule, permitted specific functions to be attributed to each

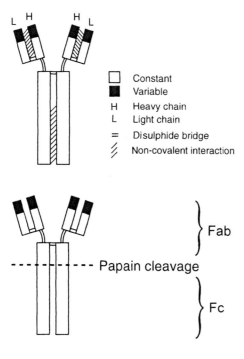

Constant
Variable
H   Heavy chain
L   Light chain
=   Disulphide bridge
// Non-covalent interaction

Papain cleavage

Fab

Fc

Figure 4.2 *The B-cell receptor for antigen (BCR), also known as immunoglobulin (Ig) or antibody (AB)*

Figure 4.3 *Enzymatic cleavage of immunoglobulin molecules yielded Fc fractions (crystallizable, hence similar in all antibodies) and Fab fractions (non-cystallizable, could bind two molecules of antigen per immunoglobulin molecule)*

When Porter and colleagues were doing their pioneering work on Ig, their source was Ig found as a plasma protein (globulin) secreted from B lymphocytes. That is how the name of Ig was derived, even though it was originally called gammaglobulin – a reference to its mobility on electrophoretic gels. Such proteins were readily accessible using techniques of the 1960s. It was not until the late 1970s and 1980s that the study of molecules present on cell surfaces became possible. This is one reason why the structure and function of the T cell receptor for antigen (TCR) was not understood until so very recently. If the plasma protein work on Ig had not been done first, it is highly likely that the name Ig would not have emerged. Rather, it is likely that 'B cell receptor for antigen (BCR)' would have become the more common term.

region of the Ig. Edelman shared the Nobel Prize with Porter. The structure suggested by these early basic biochemical techniques was later confirmed by more sophisticated techniques such as X-ray crystallography.

The Ig molecule has distinct regions that relate to different functions. The **antigen binding region (Fab)** binds specifically to antigen and each antibody has two antigen binding sites. In practice, the number of interactions possible is influenced by the hinge region that controls the degree of flexibility within the antibody molecule.

The number of different antibody molecules in an individual is enormous, perhaps up to 10^{11}. The reason for this very great diversity is the need to bind specifically to such a vast range of different antigens that may be encountered. Specificity is determined by the sequence of amino acids in the Fab region.

- Each different epitope is recognized by a different antibody. This is known as **antibody diversity**.
- Different antibodies have different sequences of amino acids in the Fab region, i.e. **the variable (V) region**.
- Amino acid sequences in regions of Ig molecules that do not interact with antigen are very similar in all antibodies. These are known as **constant (C) regions**.

It has been found that the differences in amino acid sequence between one antibody and another are not distributed evenly along the protein chain but are concentrated into short regions known as 'hot-spots' or **complementarity determining regions (CDR)**. Remembering again that antibody *in vivo* is a globular protein, we see the need for the CDR to be on the external surface of the molecule, i.e. where those amino acids can actually interact with the epitope.

The Fc portions of antibodies contain highly conserved amino acid sequences. This is the reason why the Fc fraction, when it is enzymatically cleaved from the rest of the Ig molecule, is crystallizable. The Fc portion is not involved in antigen binding but functions to anchor Ig molecules on the surface of cells that carry specific **Fc receptors**, e.g. monocytes and macrophages. Antibody molecules on the surface of an antigen serve as opsonins (Chapter 3) because phagocytes bind to them via their Fc receptors (Figure 4.4).

The physical nature of the binding between antibody and antigen is similar to that seen with other protein–protein interactions. Ideas used to explain the binding more precisely have focused upon complementary shapes, i.e. an antigen that 'fits' nicely into a space on the Ig molecule, or 'lock and key' imagery similar to that used to visualize enzyme–substrate interactions.

The many different antigens to which the immune system is exposed occur in varied micro-environments within the host. It is appropriate then that there are different classes of Ig each with

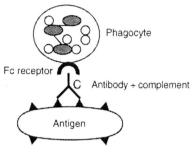

Figure 4.4 *Fc receptors on leukocytes bind to immunoglobulin molecules via their Fc regions*

Figure 4.5 *Characteristics of immunoglobulin isotypes and subtypes*

Isotype	Heavy chain	Mol. wt (kDa)	Structure	Conc. in human plasma (g/L)
IgM	μ	800	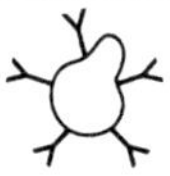	0.5–2.0
IgG1	γ1	150		5.0–12.0
IgG2	γ2	150		2.0–6.0
IgG3	γ3	165		0.5–1.0
IgG4	γ4	150		0.1–1.0
IgA1	α1	160		0.5–3.0
IgA2	α2	385	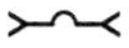	0.0–0.5
IgD	δ	170		<0.5
IgE	ε	190		<0.001

special characteristics. Figure 4.5 details the characteristics of the five major Ig classes, known as antibody **isotypes**, and their known sub-classes (subtypes):

- Isotypes: IgA, IgG, IgM, IgD, IgE
- Subtypes: IgA1, IgA2
             IgG1, IgG2, IgG3, IgG4

The heavy chains of antibodies of a particular isotype are different from those of other isotypes. Within one isotype, all subtypes have similar heavy chains.

The T cell receptor for antigen

The T cell receptor for antigen (TCR) occurs on the surface of mature T cells where it is closely associated with the CD3 molecule.

It is important to note that the isotype of an antibody does not determine its antigen binding specificity. Two antibodies of different isotype may, in fact, be specific for the same antigen. The practical rationale for this is that one antigen may be exposed to the body in different ways and the body must be able to respond effectively in each case, e.g. an antigen that enters the body through a cut blood vessel will be bound by IgG which is the predominant Ig isotype in the bloodstream. The same antigen, if it is ingested, will be bound by IgA which predominates within the gut.

Figure 4.6 *The T cell receptor for antigen (TCR) is a heterodimer comprised of either α, β or γ, δ peptide chains. On T cell surfaces it is expressed in association with CD3*

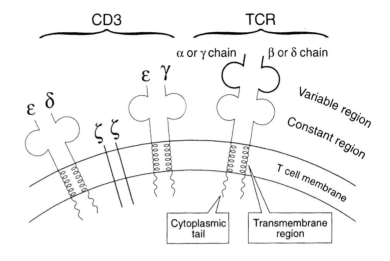

TCR and CD3 make up a group of molecules called the α, β, γ, δ and ζ (zeta) chains (Figure 4.6). The structure and function of the TCR were not elucidated until the late 1980s, indeed quite a lot of what is known has been inferred from molecular biological studies on TCR genes rather than resulting from direct biochemical analysis. The TCR bears many structural similarities to Ig, being a member of the Ig gene superfamily. It is a heterodimer comprising either an α and a β chain or a γ and a δ chain. No other combinations of the peptide chains are found. Like Ig, the TCR molecule has constant (C) and variable (V) regions, the latter being organized into CDRs.

The relationship between TCR structure and function was questioned for many years before structural information became available. It was known already that T cells could not interact with native antigen, but only with antigen that had been processed and presented in association with a 'self' MHC molecule (see below). Hence the TCR had to interact with both antigen (or epitope to be precise) and MHC molecule. Competing theories proposed were (i) that the T cell used two separate receptors for epitope and MHC and (ii) that a single receptor could interact with both molecules simultaneously. In time the latter hypothesis was shown to be correct (Figure 4.7).

The TCR itself must function in two very different ways:

- it must interact with MHC + antigen at the cell surface;
- it must transmit signals into the T cell cytoplasm so that the T cell can respond.

The second of these functions involves the cytoplasmic tails of the peptide chains that comprise the TCR-CD3 complex. The ζ chain in particular contains amino acid sequences close to its cytoplasmic terminus that can interact directly with other cytoplasmic proteins.

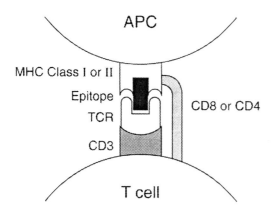

Figure 4.7 *T cells interact with antigen-presenting cells (APC). TCR recognize antigen as peptide epitope bound to self MHC*

Such interactions initiate secondary signalling pathways that transmit messages from the cell membrane to the nucleus.

Major Histocompatibility Complex antigens

This group of cell surface molecules is commonly referred to as Major Histocompatibility Complex (MHC) antigens. In order to avoid any confusion, it is important to understand fully the definition of the word 'antigen' that is given at the start of this chapter.

In contrast to Ig and TCR, it was the existence of the MHC genes that was first discovered, with determination of the structure and function of the cell surface molecules (antigens) coming very much later. The reason for this is the involvement of the MHC in transplant rejection. Simple experiments carried out in the 1940s had shown that the ability to accept or reject a transplanted organ depended very much on the genetic similarity of the organ donor and recipient. The gene locus responsible is the MHC.

The MHC antigens are not solely concerned with transplant rejection. They play significant roles in the regulation of normal acquired immune responses. There are three separate classes of MHC genes, consequently three classes of MHC antigens. The classes differ in structure, function and the cell types on which they occur.

- Class I MHC antigens occur on the surfaces of all nucleated cells and platelets.
- Class II MHC antigens occur only on cells that are closely involved with immune responses (Table 4.2). The number of molecules of an MHC antigen expressed on a cell may be altered by the presence of cytokines, e.g. IFN-γ upregulates MHC Class II expression.
- Class III MHC antigens are a diverse group of molecules that serve a wide variety of functions in the immune system, e.g.

The MHC system in humans is sometimes called the human leukocyte antigen (HLA) system. This reflects the initial incorrect assumption that MHC antigens are only expressed on leukocytes. The system in mice is known as H-2. Much of the information we have on the MHC system in humans derives from experiments in mice and other animal where deliberate inbreeding or cross-breeding is possible.

The range of different MHC antigens was discovered using the technique of serology. In this, serum from one person would react with the leukocytes from any other person who did not carry the same MHC antigens. The addition of complement would cause lysis of the leukocytes so the result could be visualized. If both the serum donor and leukocyte donor shared the same MHC antigens then lysis would not occur. This approach limits the detection of MHC antigens only to those for which an antiserum is available; hence there probably are many more different variants yet to be discovered.

Table 4.2 *Cell types where MHC Class II antigens are expressed*

B cells
Macrophages
Macrophage-like cells including:
  dendritic cells,
  Langerhans cells,
  Kupffer cells,
  glial cells,
  alveolar macrophages,
  peritoneal macrophages,
  kidney mesangial cells
Endothelial cells
Activated T cells

cytokines. Class III molecules will not be considered further at this stage.

Class I and II MHC molecules differ somewhat in structure (Figure 4.8). The principal difference is that Class I molecules comprise a single polypeptide chain but are complexed with a small protein produced by the liver and kidney and known as β_2-microglobulin. Class II antigens have two chains, α and β.

Antigen processing and presentation

The function of MHC antigens in the normal immune response is to **present** antigen to T cells via their TCR. T cells are unable to recognize antigen directly and can only participate in responses following appropriate presentation of antigen that has also been

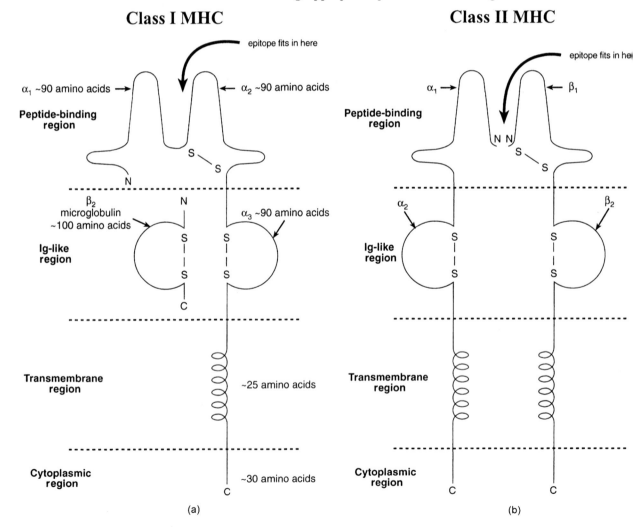

Figure 4.8 *The structures of (a) MHC Class I and (b) MHC Class II antigens*

processed. This phenomenon is known as **MHC restriction** and is one of the most important fundamental characteristics of the immune system.

Figure 4.8 shows that the part of the MHC Class I and Class II molecules in contact with the peptide antigen is the peptide binding groove. It is essential that there is tight binding between MHC antigen and peptide. The bound peptides are short, approximately nine amino acids long. For Class I in particular the peptide must fit in the groove. For Class II the size restriction is not so crucial so the peptide may overhang to either side of the MHC molecule. The bound peptides are derived from antigen and are being presented to T cells.

The next thing is to understand how antigens, most of which are, of course, much larger than nine amino acids long, are processed so that they fit the criteria for MHC presentation. The antigens that are presented by the different MHC classes are derived from different sources. Diagrams showing the pathways to presentation taken by endogenous antigen (on Class I) and exogenous antigen (on Class II) are presented in Figure 4.9. In each case the binding of epitope stabilizes the MHC antigen so allowing it to survive on the cell surface until an interaction with TCR takes place.

One interesting feature of the MHC Class I-mediated antigen presentation deserves special comment. Class I binds to endogenous epitope, i.e. peptides synthesized within the host cell. The majority of these peptides will be host molecules therefore MHC Class I antigens frequently present 'self' on the cell surface. The rationale for this is:

- To provide a mechanism through which a cell can indicate to its external environment the type of peptides that it is synthesizing. As all nucleated cells carry MHC Class I molecules, all cells capable of synthesizing protein have this 'display' facility.
- There is no mechanism by which MHC antigens can determine what is 'self' and what is 'non-self'.

The relevance of having so many different MHC antigen variants should now be becoming clear. Each separate MHC antigen differs from all the others, albeit only slightly, in its amino acid sequence and hence the shape of the antigen binding groove. Each MHC molecule can bind only to a limited range of peptide epitopes. Everybody needs to respond to many different epitopes so it is important that we express lots of different MHC antigens. Each antigen, for example a bacterium, is processed into many different epitopes but some of these will be presented, i.e. the immunodominant epitopes. Natural selection would work against an individual who lacked MHC antigens capable of presenting some of the epitopes from common dangerous pathogens so we can all

Antigen processing is the conversion of an antigen into a form in which it can be recognized by T cells. Antigen presentation is the process by which certain cells in the body (antigen-presenting cells, APCs) express antigen (as individual epitopes) on their cell surface in a form recognizable by T cells. As all nucleated cells and platelets carry MHC Class I, all cells function as APCs for endogenous antigen. The few cell types that carry MHC Class II molecules can present both endogenous and exogenous antigen. These are termed 'professional' APCs.

The use of protein chemistry techniques has allowed exploration of the question 'Which MHC antigens present which epitopes?'. By X-ray crystallography, complexes of MHC with bound epitope are isolated; 'empty' MHC antigen is unstable so is unlikely to survive the isolation procedure. The peptide and MHC can then be separated and sequenced giving a combination of both conformational (X-ray) and biochemical (sequence) data.

The process known as epitope mapping involves identification of the presented epitopes from a particular antigen. This can be very useful in designing vaccines. Vaccines which contain replicas of the immunodominant epitopes are likely to be presented and so immune responses can be initiated in the absence of the 'natural' antigen.

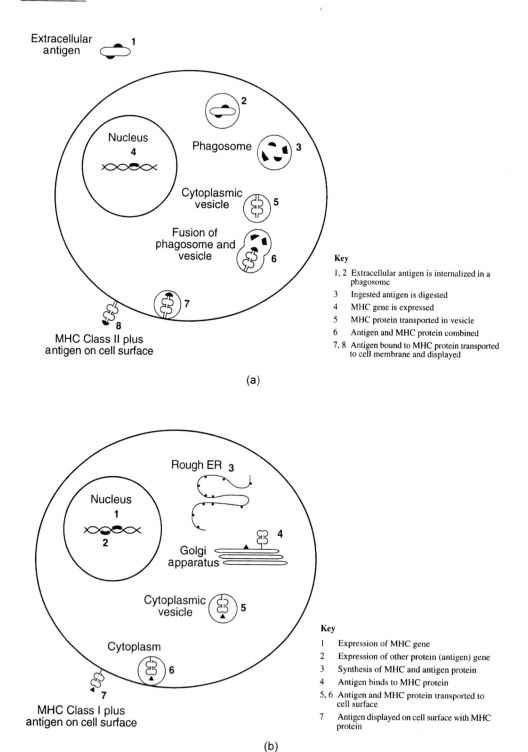

Figure 4.9   *The pathways to presentation involving (a) endogenous antigen (on MHC Class I) and (b) exogenous antigen (on MHC Class II)*

present sufficient epitopes to initiate the most important protective responses.

Genes encoding cell surface molecules involved in acquired immune responses

While TCR, Ig and MHC share protein structural similarities, the organization of their genes shows greater variation. In general, TCR and Ig genes operate in a similar fashion while MHC genes are different.

Immunoglobulin (Ig) genes

A serious question in immunology prior to the era of molecular biology techniques was: 'Are antibodies with the right antigen specificity made in response to the presence of antigen or can the antibodies exist independently of antigen?'. An early theory which has been very helpful in understanding what probably happens is **Burnet's clonal selection hypothesis** (Figure 4.10). This proposes

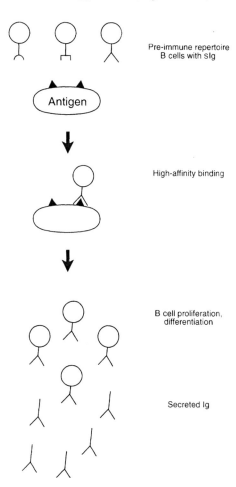

Pre-immune repertoire
B cells with sIg

Antigen

High-affinity binding

B cell proliferation, differentiation

Secreted Ig

Figure 4.10 *Burnet's clonal selection hypothesis. The pre-immune repertoire is changed following encounter with antigen. The lymphocytes bearing receptors that bind to the antigen proliferate so are present in higher numbers than those that did not bind antigen*

$$\text{Affinity} = \frac{[\text{TCR} - \text{MHC}]}{[\text{TCR}][\text{MHC}]}$$

i.e. higher affinity predisposes to tight binding between TCR and MHC.

that mature lymphocytes express a wide range of receptor specificities, i.e. Ig or TCR, with slightly different variable regions – although any one mature cell expresses only one specificity. These all exist independently of antigen. The range of specificities is known as the **pre-immune repertoire**. When antigen is encountered it binds with greater or lesser affinity to the receptors. This binding leads to proliferation of the 'selected' lymphocyte to form a clone of cells bearing receptors identical to the parent lymphocyte. After the response, the cells which proliferated now predominate so the repertoire of receptor specificities has changed through encounter with antigen – one of the hallmarks of acquired responses (Chapter 5). Central to this idea is the expression of receptor specificities before antigen is encountered so they must be genetically determined. Burnet's hypothesis came remarkably close to explaining events for which there now is experimental evidence.

It has been estimated that about 10^9 or 10^{10} different Ig and TCR specificities are needed to engage strongly with all possible antigens. If Ig and TCR genes worked on the basis of one gene–one receptor specificity, this would require there to be more genes than there are in the entire human genome. We now understand that a system of gene rearrangements operates to build up about 10^{11} different specificities from a small number, about a couple of hundred, gene segments. This phenomenon is termed **V(D)J recombination**. It was originally worked out for Ig formation in maturing B cells but precisely the same principles hold true for TCR formation also.

The constant regions of Ig are expressed by single genes for each isotype, i.e. a very small number of different genes. The gene rearrangements that will be considered encode only the variable regions of the antibody molecules so we have a situation where each protein chain of the molecule is the product of more than one gene. It was 1983 before a paper, by Susumu Tonegawa (a Nobel prize-winner in 1987), explaining how Ig variable region genes are organized, was published in the journal Nature.

The genes for Ig heavy chains are found on chromosome 14 with those for light chains being on chromosomes 2 and 22. The protein chain expressed by chromosome 2 genes is called the κ (kappa) chain and that from chromosome 22 is the λ (lambda) chain. Figure 4.11 shows schematically the arrangement of Ig genes found in the human germline, i.e. the DNA, as it is found in all somatic cells except mature B cells. The reason why mature B cell DNA is different is because gene rearrangement has taken place. By contrasting the germline heavy chain sequence with the heavy chain sequence in the mature B cell (Figure 4.11), the nature of the rearrangement can be seen. From the original complete set of variable region Ig genes, a small number have been selected and brought together so that they now lie in a continuous sequence of DNA. This final sequence contains just one of the several **V (variable) genes**, one of the **D (diversity) genes** and one of the **J (joining) genes**. All other 'unused' V, D and J genes are deleted.

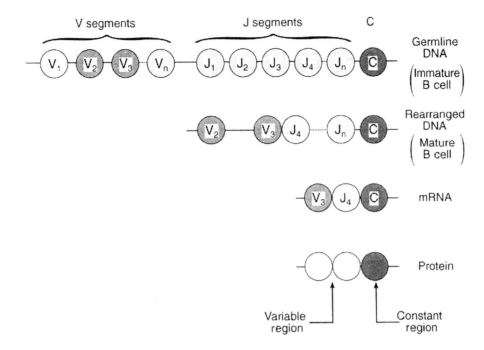

Figure 4.11 *The arrangement of Ig genes, or gene segments, found in the human germline in immature B cells is rearranged during maturation. Mature B cells can produce Ig of only a single specificity (idiotype)*

Rearrangement is considered to be a random process therefore each V, D and J gene has an equal chance of being 'selected' for the final DNA sequence. Thus many, many different VDJ combinations are possible. This is the principal source of the great diversity seen in Ig molecules.

To complete the assembly of the Ig sequence, the VDJ is complexed with a constant region gene to specify the antibody isotype. The constant region gene closest to the variable genes is μ, therefore IgM is the first isotype to be produced by a B cell (Figure 4.12). When antibody is being synthesized, the mRNA is transcribed from the rearranged DNA sequence and translated to yield a variable region peptide. In subsequent rounds of Ig synthesis, the constant region may be changed (because the complexing of variable region and constant region occurred at mRNA level) thus producing antibody of the same specificity as on the first occasion, but of different isotype. This change is regulated by T cells and by the cytokine IL-4. The phenomenon by which the antibody isotype expressed by a B cell can be changed is known as **Ig class switching** or **isotype switching**. The sequence of events described here relates to Ig gene rearrangements for heavy chains. The light chain events are similar except that D genes are absent, the variable regions being constructed only of V and J genes.

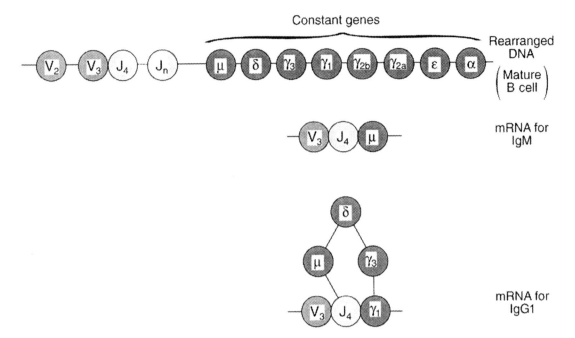

Figure 4.12 *IgM is the first isotype to be produced by a B cell when it is stimulated to respond*

The rearrangement of Ig genes is a significant source of antibody diversity, however the total number of gene combinations possible may be augmented in the following ways:

- When V gene DNA is joining with the D gene DNA, up to about three nucleotides may be lost or gained. This alters the reading frame for the triplet code. It is estimated that this increases the diversity 10-fold. Similarly, the joining of D to J introduces a 10-fold increase in variability.
- Heavy chain and light chain DNA are rearranged independently. In Ig assembly any two identical heavy chains can join with any two identical λ light chains or any two identical κ light chains (but not with one λ and one κ chain).
- There is a high frequency of somatic mutation among Ig genes. The mutation frequency may be up to 10 000 times greater than that of other genes.

The final assembly of Ig molecules includes the linking of light and heavy chains through inter-chain disulphide bridges and the addition of high-mannose carbohydrates. Before their expression on the B cell surface or their secretion, Ig molecules undergo final modifications such as the alteration of carbohydrate side-chains and the addition of other peptides, e.g. the 'J' chain of IgM (which is totally unrelated to the J gene of the variable region) (Chapter 5).

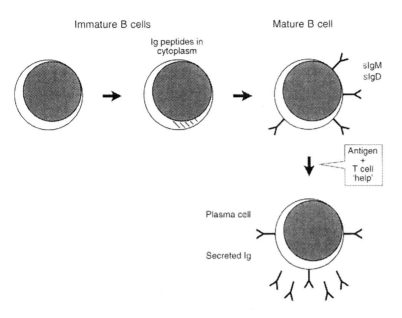

Figure 4.13 *As a B cell matures in the bone marrow, it initially produces Ig only on its surface (sIg). Following encounter with antigen, differentiation and proliferation lead to a clone of identical plasma cells that are capable of secreting Ig*

B cell maturation

As a B cell matures in the bone marrow, it initially produces Ig only on its surface (**sIg**, Figure 4.13). This sIg includes both IgM and IgD. Any B cell that fails to express surface IgD and IgM together will not be allowed to mature further but will die. At later stages, maturing cells acquire the capacity to secrete antibody while also retaining sIg. The secreted form is not just a shortened version of the sIg but is synthesized without the membrane-spanning region that anchors the sIg on the B cell surface. Both the sIg and secreted Ig from a single B cell have identical antigen specificity. This specificity does not alter throughout the lifetime of the B cell.

The very great specificity of antibody binding, and the fact that individual B cell clones produce antibody of only a single specificity, has allowed them to be exploited to great benefit in the laboratory. Antibodies are used extensively in diagnostic laboratories and in research techniques. This is because the specificity of antibodies greatly exceeds that of any chemical. A significant fraction of the world's biotechnology industry is based upon the production of monoclonal antibodies that can be designed and produced within laboratories in order to meet the needs of biomedical scientists (Chapter 10). Limited success has also been achieved using tailor-made monoclonal antibodies for *in vivo* patient treatment, however the benefits of this approach have never quite managed to live up to its promise.

TCR genes

Genes encoding the peptide chains of TCR are organized in a

manner similar to that of Ig genes and also undergo random rearrangement of the germline. Once again there are V, D, J and C genes present in the DNA for TCR protein chains. The high rate of somatic mutation that occurs in Ig genes is absent in TCR genes.

T cell maturation

It is in the stages of maturation of the T cells that major and important differences from the B cell lineage occur. These important stages take place in the thymus through **thymic processing**. Information gained from developing mouse embryos indicates that immature T cells in the thymus (**thymocytes**) rearrange TCR genes as an early event that is followed closely by TCR mRNA expression and the appearance of TCR/CD3 on the cell surface. Later, other cell surface molecules that define T cells, i.e. CD4 and CD8, begin to appear also. (Expression of molecules CD1, CD2 and CD5 is thought to precede TCR/CD3 expression.)

Once the polypeptide chains of TCR and CD3 have been stably expressed the selection of those thymocytes that will reach maturity takes place. Selection proceeds in two stages: **positive selection and negative selection**.

- Positive selection allows the survival of thymocytes bearing TCR that bind with self MHC.
- Negative selection ensures the removal of thymocytes bearing TCR that bind tightly to self MHC complexed with a self peptide.

During positive selection events thymocytes expressing both CD4 and CD8 (CD4$^+$ CD8$^+$ cells) interact with the cells of the cortical thymus (Figure 4.14). If any thymocytes bind, via their TCR, to thymic epithelial cells expressing self MHC Class I or Class II molecules, the thymocytes will receive signals allowing them to survive. Thymocytes that are unable to bind to self MHC will be deprived of survival signals and hence will die by apoptosis.

Thymocytes that survive positive selection also undergo changes that determine whether they will mature into T cells that can interact with self MHC Class I or Class II antigens.

- Thymocytes with low affinity for self MHC Class I will lose their CD4 and become CD8$^+$ T cells capable of interacting only with self MHC Class I.
- Thymocytes that interact weakly with self MHC Class II will lose their CD8 to become CD4$^+$ T cells capable of interacting only with self MHC Class II.

Negative selection is used to ensure that no T cell can mature with the ability to bind tightly to self MHC + self peptide. This is the basis of the state of **immunological tolerance** in which immune responses are not normally directed against the self.

Thymocytes that survive the selection processes leave the thymus

Immunological tolerance, specifically tolerance of self, was first demonstrated experimentally in the 1950s by Sir Peter Medawar and colleagues. Medawar shared the 1960 Nobel prize for medicine with Sir Macfarlane Burnet (see also Burnet's clonal selection hypothesis). Medawar's group worked on a skin graft (skin transplant) system in which a graft between adult mice of two different strains would be rejected. With newborn mice of the same two strains, however, leukocytes could be transferred from one strain to another without rejection. When the mice who had received the leukocytes grew up, they could accept skin grafts from the other strain. This meant that the newborn mice regarded the foreign leukocytes as being normal self components and developed tolerance to their antigens when their T cells were undergoing maturation.

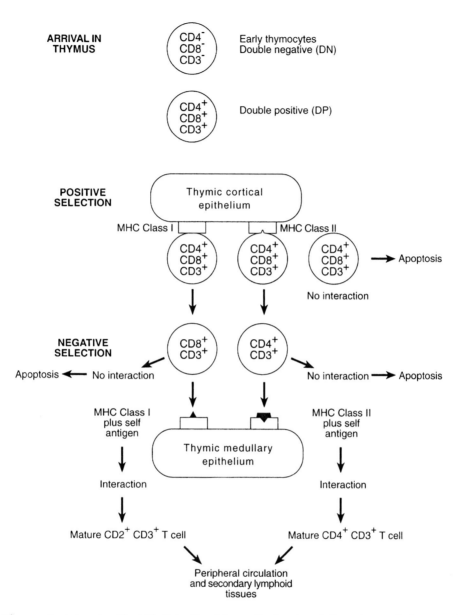

Figure 4.14 *Thymocytes interact with epithelial cells of the cortical and medullary thymus before entering the circulation as mature T cells*

and enter the peripheral circulation, moving between the circulation and secondary lymphoid tissues and participating in immune responses. Once mature, any strong interactions with MHC will induce proliferation of the T cell (i.e. the opposite to the cell death which accompanied strong interactions by thymocytes). The maturation of thymocytes appears to continue throughout life, albeit in much reduced numbers following thymic atrophy.

Major Histocompatibility Complex genes

In humans, Major Histocompatibility Complex (MHC) genes are on chromosome 6 although the gene for β_2 microglobulin is on chromosome 15. Unlike Ig and TCR molecules the wide diversity of MHC is not created by gene rearrangements, rather it is due to the extreme polymorphism of the MHC genes. The MHC genes are among the most polymorphic of all known mammalian genes, i.e. there are many, perhaps over 40, different alleles of each gene. Every few years attempts are made to draw very complex maps depicting the current state of knowledge of MHC genes. One immediately obvious feature of such maps is that many of the genes have not yet been ascribed a function and many of the protein products have not been characterized.

Each nucleated cell in a person's body expresses a pattern of MHC antigens which is genetically determined by MHC genes and is unique to that person (unless he or she has an identical twin, in which case both twins have an identical pattern). The pattern is made up of one set of gene alleles inherited from each parent, i.e. two **haplotypes**. The alleles that are expressed determine the nature of the MHC antigens and this is known as a **tissue type**.

Interaction of TCR and MHC antigens is necessary for immune responses

T cells recognize antigen via interactions of their TCR with self MHC + peptide on the surface of other cells. These other accessory cells are known as **antigen-presenting cells (APCs)**. Not every T cell can, however, interact with every self MHC + peptide complex. The pattern of interaction is:

- only T cells that carry CD8 on the cell surface can interact with MHC Class I + peptide;
- only T cells that carry CD4 on the cell surface can interact with MHC Class II + peptide.

This distinction is possible because the CD8 and CD4 molecules interact with non-polymorphic (constant) regions of the MHC Class I and MHC Class II molecules, respectively. This binding stabilizes the interaction between the APC and the T cell but it does not regulate T cell recognition of the presented antigen.

If we combine the information already given about the binding of peptide antigen with each MHC Class, and that on T cell specificities, a picture emerges of different T cells interacting with different types of antigen.

- CD8$^+$ cells bind to endogenous antigen on MHC Class I positive APC. **Endogenous antigen may be self, tumour antigen or viral antigen.**

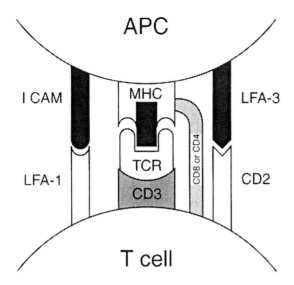

- CD4[+] T cells bind to exogenous antigen on MHC Class II positive APC. Exogenous antigen is derived from any foreign material that can exist extracellularly, e.g. bacteria, fungi, parasites, other soluble proteins and viruses that have not (yet) gained entry to normal cells.

When APCs and T cells interact via MHC–TCR, it is important that close contact between the two cells is maintained. The strength of the interaction between these two molecules appears to be insufficient so a number of other accessory molecules are employed. These molecules function in a similar way to a zipper. The strength of the multiple interactions is significantly greater than that of a single point of contact. Figure 4.15 illustrates how molecules on the APC surface are 'paired' with complementary molecules on the T cell surface. Similar accessory molecules are employed for both MHC Class I–CD8[+] interactions and MHC Class II–CD4[+] interactions. It is now known that the multiple interactions also deliver signals to the T cell. These are known as **co-stimulatory** signals and are essential for T cell activation.

Suggested further reading

Anderson, G., Moore, N.C., Owen, J.J.T. and Jenkinson, E.J. (1996) Cellular interactions in thymocyte development. *Annual Review of Immunology* **14**, 73–99.

Banchereau, J. and Steinman, R.M. (1998) Dendritic cells and the control of immunity. *Nature* **392**, 245–252.

Camacho, S.A., Kosco-Vilbois, M.H. and Berek, C. (1998) The dynamic structure of the germinal centre. *Immunology Today* **19**, 511–514.

Cantrell, D. (1996) T cell antigen receptor signal transduction pathways. *Annual Review of Immunology* **14**, 259–274.

Daeron, M. (1997) Fc receptor biology. *Annual Review of Immunology* **15**, 203–234.

Ghia, P., tenBoekel, E., Rolink, A.G. and Melchers, F. (1998) B cell development: a comparison between mouse and man. *Immunology Today* **19**, 480–485.

Kearse, K.P., Roberts, J.P., Wiest, D.L. and Singer, A. (1995) Developmental regulation of αβ T cell antigen receptor assembly in CD4$^+$CD8$^+$ thymocytes. *Bioessays* **17**, 1049–1054.

Pamer, E. and Cresswell, P. (1998) Mechanisms of MHC Class I-restricted antigen processing. *Annual Review of Immunology* **16**, 323–358.

Porter, R.R. (1959) The hydrolysis of rabbit γ-globulin and antibodies by crystalline papain. *Biochemical Journal* **73**, 119.

Rasko, I. and Downes, C.S. (1995) Genes in Medicine. London: Chapman and Hall.

Tonegawa, S. (1983) Somatic generation of antibody diversity. *Nature* **302**, 575–581.

Watts, C. (1997) Capture and processing of exogenous antigens for presentation on MHC molecules. *Annual Review of Immunology* **15**, 821–850.

Self-assessment questions

1. How many immunoglobulin domains occur in each of the following molecules: CD4, CD8, TCR, MHC Class I, MHC Class II, IgE?
2. Distinguish between the Fab and Fc regions of an Ig molecule.
3. In theory, how many antigenic determinants could be bound by a single IgM molecule?
4. If the expression $(\lambda_2\kappa_2)_2$ describes the protein constituents of an IgA dimer, write two such expressions to describe IgG (ignoring the existence of IgG subclasses).
5. Name one cell type that does not express MHC Class I antigen.
6. What information do you have from this chapter to prove that Ig gene rearrangement occurs at the DNA level and not at the RNA or protein level?
7. List three structural or functional differences between MHC Class I and MHC Class II molecules.
8. List at least three cell surface molecules that could be used to define a T cell that would interact with virus antigen presented by an APC.
9. Define immunological tolerance and state how it arises.
10. What is the principal type of chemical interaction that maintains the shape of Ig and related molecules?

Key Concepts and Facts

Immunoglobulin (Ig)
- Ig, or antibody, is produced by B cells as surface Ig or in secreted form.

- The Ig molecule binds to antigen. Different Ig molecules can bind different antigens because of highly variable amino acid sequences in their Fab regions.

- Antibody diversity is due principally to random gene rearrangements whereby a small number of Ig genes can give rise to some 10^{11} different antigen binding specificities.

- There are five principal Ig classes (isotypes) with varying characteristics, functions and sites of occurrence in the body. This allows for slightly different interactions to take place with different antigens in different *in vivo* environments.

T-cell Receptor for Antigen (TCR)
- TCR occurs on the surface of T cells and its structure is similar to Ig.

- TCR cannot bind to native antigen directly but only to antigen that has been processed and presented in association with self MHC antigens on cell surfaces. This is MHC restriction.

- TCR diversity results from random rearrangements of genes. Immature T cells then undergo selection in the thymus to remove non-functional T cells or those with TCR that would bind tightly to self MHC + self peptide.

Major Histocompatibility Complex (MHC) Antigens
- MHC antigens regulate the rejection or acceptance of transplanted tissue and also function in normal immune responses.

- Class I MHC antigens occur on all nucleated cells and platelets. Class II MHC antigens occur only on cells closely associated with the immune system.

- Class I MHC antigens bind and present endogenous antigen that is recognized by $CD8^+$ T cells. Class II MHC antigens bind and present exogenous antigen that is recognized by $CD4^+$ T cells.

- Different MHC antigen variants arise through a high degree of polymorphism at MHC gene loci.

Chapter 5
Acquired immune responses

Learning objectives

After studying this chapter you should confidently be able to:

List the principal characteristics of acquired immune responses.

Discuss the concepts of immunological specificity and immunological memory.

Describe the interactions of antigen-presenting cells and lymphocytes, in the presence of antigen, that initiate responses.

Describe the role of cytokines in the initiation of immune responses.

Describe the sequence of events that comprise acquired immune responses.

Discuss how acquired immune responses may vary in different parts of the body.

Discuss the interaction of the immune system with the nervous and endocrine systems.

Consider that each person who was immunized as a child against a range of diseases is an example of both immunological specificity and memory. The response against an antigen delivered in a vaccine protects against one form of infectious disease. For protection against another disease, another antigen must be delivered to the person. Different antigens may be delivered simultaneously (in a 'combined' vaccine) but the response against each one is specific.

Immunizations done at a few weeks of life confer protection for many years, or a whole lifetime in some cases. This demonstrates memory.

Characteristics of acquired immune responses

In Chapter 4 all of the major 'characters', i.e. cells and molecules, that play a role in acquired immune responses were introduced. In addition, those events that must precede a response, i.e. antigen processing and presentation, were described. Once all the necessary components and conditions are in place, a response can be initiated. The response will have some very special characteristics that form the basis of the distinction between natural and acquired responses. The characteristics are specificity and memory.

Specificity

The specificity of acquired immune responses is exceptionally important. This importance is underlined by the complexity of the biological features that regulate specificity (Chapter 4). **An acquired response against one epitope is unique to that epitope.**

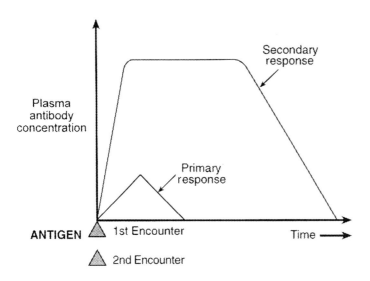

Figure 5.1 *Primary and secondary immune responses differ in their time course and extent. The primary response is slower and less effective than the swifter, stronger secondary response*

Figure 5.1 shows the results of a simple hypothetical experiment that illustrates these features. The initial response to an antigen, the **primary response,** is relatively slow. This may be attributed to the number of stages that must be accomplished. Subsequent exposure to the same antigen induces **secondary responses** that are swifter and more powerful than the primary response. This is seen in the case of infectious diseases that normally occur just once in a person's lifetime, e.g. measles or chicken pox. During the initial bout of disease, when the person is most likely to be ill, the primary response takes place. If the person is exposed to the same disease at a later time, they may display only very mild symptoms or none at all. Immunization is effective in precisely the same way. The effective secondary response does not allow the infection to take hold as the infectious agent is eliminated rapidly.

The primary and secondary immune responses may be distinguished as follows:

- the secondary response is faster and antibody levels are much higher;
- the secondary response persists longer than the primary;
- IgG is the predominant antibody in the primary response while IgM dominates in the secondary;
- the average affinity of antibodies for antigen is higher in the secondary response.

In the case of immunization, it is sometimes necessary to receive booster injections, i.e. re-exposure to the antigen, in order to maintain the effectiveness of the response. Immunization with a specific vaccine is currently necessary against each different infectious disease that we wish to be immune to. The development of a vaccine that would confer immunity to a range of diseases simultaneously is currently a goal of vaccine biotechnologists.

The nature and extent of an immune response is determined primarily by antigen. At the most basic level, the presence of antigen may be regarded as the 'on–off' switch, i.e. if antigen is not present, a response cannot take place. Other more subtle factors are also important:

- The nature of the antigen. Endogenous antigen stimulates responses through MHC Class I presentation to $CD8^+$ T cells while exogenous antigen causes MHC Class II presentation to $CD4^+$ T cells (Chapter 4).
- Degree of difference from self. In general, self antigens elicit tolerance, not response, while non-self antigens stimulate response. Some foreign (non-self) antigens may, however, resemble self so the response is likely to be weak.
- Antigen size. Larger antigens are more likely to stimulate responses.
- Antigen dose. Below a threshold dose, a response is not initiated. Excessively high concentrations of antigen may also predispose to less effective responses.
- The route of entry of the antigen to the body. Antigens that enter via the bloodstream are likely to be cleared from the circulation into the spleen where responses will take place. Conversely, antigens that are ingested may be taken to the lymph nodes before a response takes place or they may induce tolerance instead of response through encounters with gut lymphocytes.

The appropriate initiation of immune responses is critically dependent on the T cell recognition of processed and presented antigen. Once these events have occurred, the next step will be either response or non-response (**tolerance**). Response is the outcome only if T cells can interact with high affinity with the presented epitope on self-MHC antigen. If thymic processing of T cells has proceeded in its normal, efficient manner, the only T cells capable of this high-affinity binding will be those with TCR specific for self MHC in combination with foreign epitopes. The recognition events are shown in Figure 5.2. The cell surface events are seen to be accompanied by cytokine production. The release of the cytokines and the appropriate responses by the target cells are necessary regulatory events. The combination of intercellular interaction and responses to cytokines causes the **activation of T cells**.

> The activation of T cells in response to antigen is the stimulus for a wide array of immune responses. It is critically important that this activation occurs only on appropriate occasions, i.e. only in response to non-self, because a response directed against self can cause significant damage to normal host tissues. The biological 'investment' in T cells is considerable. Some 95% of all T cells that are produced by the bone marrow may be eliminated during thymic processing. The 'pay-back' of ensuring the avoidance of anti-self responses makes it all worthwhile.

> Normally, all cases in which self epitopes are presented on self-MHC will result in tolerance. This is the important outcome of the thymic deletion of potentially self-reactive T cells. The T cell will not bind strongly to self-MHC carrying self peptide therefore no response ensues, i.e. there is self tolerance. When a non-self epitope is presented, the T cell can respond.

The nature of acquired responses

The response that follows from T cell activation depends on the nature of the T cell that is activated (Figure 5.3).

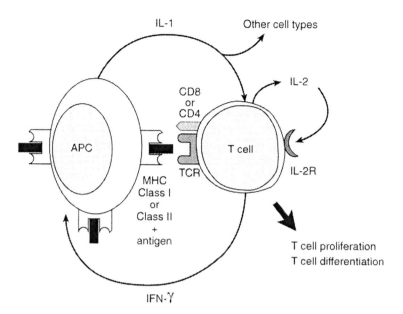

Figure 5.2 *T cell recognition of antigen presented in association with MHC on an APC. The APC produces IL-1 which stimulates the expression of IL-2 receptors on T cells. These receptors are necessary to allow the response to IL-2 to take place. The stimulated T cell also produces IFNγ that feeds back to the APC, upregulating MHC Class II antigen expression*

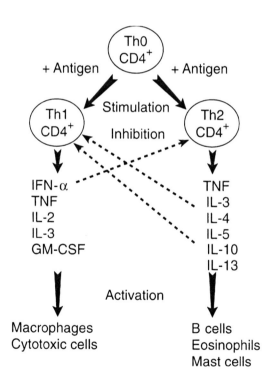

Figure 5.3 *Cells are directed both by antigen and by cytokines to develop functions that deal effectively with different types of exogenous antigen. Th1 cells favour cell-mediated responses while Th2 responses are antibody-mediated*

- A CD8$^+$ T cell will initiate a **cell-mediated response** known as a **cytotoxic response**.
- A CD4$^+$ T cell will initiate an **antibody-mediated response**, also termed a **humoral response**.

Cytotoxic responses

Following activation of CD8$^+$ T cells, **proliferation and differentiation** occur. The responding T cell undergoes several rounds of mitosis to form a clone of T cells with TCR identical to the initial cell which engaged with MHC + epitope. Many cells in that clone will differentiate into **cytotoxic, or cytolytic, T cells (CTL)** capable of directly lysing virally-infected or tumour cells, others will persist as memory cells. The differentiation requires not only the cytokine IL-2 and IFN-γ but probably also IL-4, IL-6, IL-7 and IL-12. The source of these cytokines may be CD4$^+$ T cells, however that is currently unclear as some experiments appear to show CD8$^+$ cell differentiation into CTLs in the absence of CD4$^+$ cells. The CD4$^+$ T cell that are thought to assist CD8$^+$ cells are known as **helper T cells**.

The CTLs function by destroying cells that contain non-self. This includes tumour cells and virally infected cells. It is important to note that, in a particular response, CTLs will target only cells displaying non-self epitope identical to that on the cell that was originally recognized by a CD8$^+$ cell.

There are two distinct killing mechanisms that CTLs employ. The first of these is a pore-forming protein system called **perforin (or cytolysin)**. The second type of killing involves a cytokine called **lymphotoxin (LT)**. There is a significant degree of structural similarity between LT and the pro-inflammatory cytokine TNF-α so an alternate, but infrequently used, name for LT is TNF-β. Both the perforin and LT are stored in the CTL within cytoplasmic granules. When the CTL and target cell engage, the granules migrate to the side of the CTL that is closest to the target. The CTL then degranulates and the toxic contents are released. This release causes the perforins to encounter the higher calcium concentration of extracellular medium and to respond by polymerization to form polyperforin. Polyperforin is a pore-forming molecule that inserts itself into the lipid bilayer of the target and the cell dies in the same manner as cells attacked by the membrane attack complex (MAC) of complement (Chapter 3). On exposure to LT, the target cell dies by apoptosis. The precise mechanism of this killing is poorly understood. The mode of cell killing by CTLs seems to be very efficient and non-hazardous to the host because:

- the lethal molecules are delivered precisely to the target so there is little risk of causing damage to adjacent normal cells;
- the CTL themselves are not damaged.

Destruction of a virally infected cell might be thought to be potentially hazardous as it could cause the liberation of virus particles that would then be free to infect other adjacent host cells. This undesirable consequence is avoided by the secretion of IFN-γ from the CTL. Some of the functions of this IFN-γ are:

- To induce an **anti-viral state**. This means that the interferon has been inserted into the outer membrane of adjacent cells. Viruses are unable to infect cells that are protected in this way. Other interferons, α and β, which are components of the natural immune response, are also produced during viral infections. Natural interferons strongly promote the anti-viral state.
- To activate macrophages. The macrophages phagocytose free (extracellular) virus particles.

The IFN-γ may also allow interaction with other elements of the immune response and so lead to antibody production and complement activation. Both of these molecules can then act as opsonins to enhance phagocytosis of viruses.

Antibody-mediated responses

If the T cell that recognized the presented antigen was a $CD4^+$ T cell, once again some proliferation and differentiation will take place. Some cells will become memory cells while others will interact with B cells. This interaction induces B cell proliferation and differentiation. Most of these B cells differentiate to form a clone of antibody-secreting **plasma cells** while others become memory cells. The interaction of activated T cells with B cells is antigen specific which means that the B cells induced to proliferate will be those that can recognize the same antigen as that which was presented to the T cell. The antibodies secreted will be able to bind to the antigen. This process of passing on a message from T cells to B cells is complex, particularly so because B cell receptors (Ig) recognize antigen in its native state rather than the processed version which stimulated the T cell. It is important that the secreted antibodies also recognize native antigen because that is what they must interact with following their secretion.

Antibody-mediated responses are designed to deal with a vast array of foreign materials. The responses are very well 'tailored' to cope with the particular antigen that initially induced the T cell activation. This tailoring is not so clearly seen at the earliest stages of a response on initial contact with the antigen, but rather it develops as a response progresses.

Once B cells are activated and antibodies are secreted from plasma cells, the process of **affinity maturation** commences. This is also a mechanism to increase the efficiency of an immune response that is already underway. The binding affinity of the population of antibodies, with antigen, is low at the start of the response but gradually improves. This is a feature that can be best understood by thinking about antigenic determinants (epitopes) as different shapes, as illustrated by Burnet's clonal selection hypothesis (Chapter 4). In the primary response the epitope that stimulated the response can be bound by antibodies of several different complementary 'shapes'. Some shapes bind more tightly than

> At this point it should be becoming clear why it is that T cells are considered to be the central, most important, regulatory cell type in the immune system. It does not matter that B cells which rearranged Ig genes to express potentially self-reactive Ig idiotypes were not deleted. They will never be activated because the corresponding T cells were deleted in the thymus.

others, i.e. they are of higher affinity. Gradually the amount of antigen in the system will be reduced so only the antibodies of highest affinity, whether secreted or on B-cell surfaces, will have a chance of binding antigen. When surface Ig is not being bound by antigen, the B cell dies by apoptosis. Therefore, in the secondary response, those B cells producing antibodies with the highest affinity will predominate and the production of lower affinity antibodies will be reduced. Affinity maturation is also fuelled by the very high rate of somatic mutation known to occur in Ig V region genes. This increases the possible range of antibody specificities with a consequently greater chance of producing an antibody of very high affinity. Of course the mutation can also lead to antibodies of lower affinity but these will not bind antibody so the B cells that produced them will be eliminated.

Antibody-mediated immune responses are not terminated when antibody binds to the target. The destruction of the target is caused by complement that is activated via the classical pathway, attached to the hinge region of the antibody molecules (Chapter 4). The target is now coated with antibody and complement fragments, i.e. it is opsonized. It is finally removed by phagocytes, attracted by the release of complement anaphylatoxins, which bind to the target via Fc receptors for antibody and complement receptors.

Figure 5.3 indicates how CD4$^+$ cells are directed both by antigen and by cytokines to develop functions that deal effectively with different types of exogenous antigen. It should be clear from the diagram that CD4$^+$ cells are capable of activating a wide range of other effector cell types. Some of those cells may be considered to be part of natural immune responses however, in reality, there is no real boundary between natural and acquired responses. This T cell mediated central coordination of many different aspects of immune responses is a significant strength of the human immune system. The existence in humans of **Th1 and Th2** subsets of CD4$^+$ cells was questioned for many years. One reason for the lack of acceptance of the concept was that the subsets cannot (yet) be defined on the basis of cell surface markers to which labelled 'tags' might be attached. The ability to secrete a particular collection of cytokines is the only defining feature and this can only be assessed *in vitro*.

Responses to T cell independent antigen

The vast majority of acquired immune responses are directed against antigens that are presented to T cells via self MHC. We express this by saying that most antigens are **T-dependent** and that the T cells are **MHC-restricted**. There is also a small group of antigens which are recognized directly by B cells leading to antibody-mediated responses. These are mostly carbohydrate antigens consisting of repeating sequences of a single sugar monomer (Figure 5.4). This type of molecule is only found on the outer wall of some bacteria, never on mammalian cells. It is safe therefore

B cell

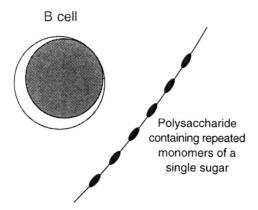

Polysaccharide
containing repeated
monomers of a
single sugar

Figure 5.4 *T-independent antigens are mostly carbohydrate (polysaccharide) antigens consisting of repeating sequences of a single sugar monomer*

for B cells to react independently against such antigens as the responses could not be directed against self.

Intracellular signalling in lymphocytes

Up to this point we have considered the interaction between lymphocytes and antigen only from the perspective of cell-surface and extracellular events. We need now to extend our understanding of the regulation of the lymphocyte response by considering intracellular changes that are brought about by signals travelling from the cell surface. This is known as intracellular signalling. It is important to realize that cell surface molecules have roles in transmitting signals into the cell. For example, some of the TCR/ CD3 subunits are clearly involved in physical interaction with MHC–peptide complexes while other subunits transmit signals, through their cytoplasmic regions, to intracellular second messenger systems and thence to the nucleus. Our understanding of intracellular signalling that leads to T cell activation has increased considerably in recent years.

Once TCR has bound to self MHC + antigen, intracellular signalling commences with a cascade of enzyme-catalysed events (Figure 5.5). Remember that the TCR and other cell surface molecules of the Ig superfamily each contain a C-terminal region that extends into the T cell cytoplasm. This region is not just an inert anchor. It also contains enzyme activity, most commonly tyrosine kinase activity. Other cytoplasmic proteins interact with the cytoplasmic tails and so a cascade of phosphorylation–dephosphorylation events can be initiated.

It is now known that intracellular activation signals generated within T cells are similar to many of those used in other non-lymphocyte cell types, i.e. phosphorylation, hydrolysis of inositol phosphates and alteration of intracellular calcium and protein kinase C (PKC) activities. The transition time between the T cell surface and the nucleus is a couple of minutes. After this time the

Our understanding of the central role of T cells has taken a long time to emerge. During the nineteenth century battles raged between the 'cellularists' and 'humoralists' (those who believed in an immune system that existed as non-cellular components). The discovery in the 1890s that immune serum (i.e. serum containing antibodies) could protect against diphtheria and tetanus swung opinion in the definite direction of the humoralists, most of whom were French. The German, or Prussian, dominated cellularists retaliated and this has even been cited as one of the reasons that perpetuated the animosity of the Franco–Prussian war and led to the outbreak of the First World War. Thus a 'chemical' perspective on Immunology dominated well into the twentieth century.

Figure 5.5 *Signals generated at a T cell surface are transmitted to the T cell nucleus. One of the principal events is protein phosphorylation*

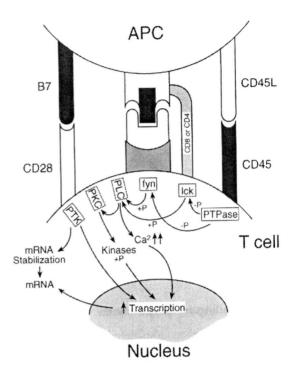

transcription of T cell genes may be detected. Important mediators in the signalling pathway are transcription factors. These include nuclear factor kappa B (NFκB), a cytoplasmic transcription factor that is activated when released from its inhibitor, IκB. The active NFκB translocates to the nucleus and binds with an appropriate part of the DNA, e.g. the promoter region of the IL-2 gene. This binding increases many-fold transcription of the IL-2 gene such that elevated IL-2 mRNA, as well as mRNA for other cytokines, appears about 1 hour following TCR–MHC interaction. The production of IL-2 is of such major significance for T cell activation that there are several different pathways leading to its transcription. Other transcription factors that are involved include NF-AT and AP-1.

Intracellular signalling is probably not initiated by TCR alone. In Chapter 4 the need for multiple interactions to take place between T cell and antigen-presenting cell (APC) surfaces was discussed. While the analogy of a 'zipper' has been used to illustrate the effect of this multiple binding, it is insufficient. The binding of the various other complementary molecules is thought also to generate signals within the T cell that direct subsequent gene expression. The molecules B7 on professional APCs and CD28 on T cells are one example of a complementary pair whose binding generates intracellular signals that are necessary for T cell activation. Molecules such as B7 and CD28 are known as co-stimulators. Their interaction alone, in the absence of TCR binding to MHC + antigen, would be insufficient to cause T cell activation.

The cytokine IL-2 was originally termed T cell growth factor. This cytokine demonstrates autocrine action. Once TCR interaction with MHC and antigen has occurred, the T cells are both the source of the cytokine, and the responder cell population.

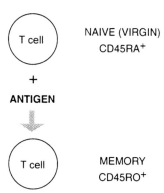

Figure 5.6 *The CD45 molecule is altered when the T cell is activated by encounter with antigen. Most naive T cells are CD45RA$^+$ while those that have encountered antigen generally are CD45RO$^+$*

Immunological memory

While there can be no doubt about the existence of immunological memory, its cellular and molecular mechanisms remain somewhat obscure. Our current concept involves an initial contact with antigen that generates antigen-specific T cells and B cells that persist in the circulation, i.e. antigen-specific memory cells. On subsequent encounters with the same antigen, the memory cells are rapidly re-stimulated. The precise lifespan of a lymphocyte has proved hard to determine, however it is perfectly feasible for the memory cells to undergo mitosis to produce identical daughter cells that retain the 'memory' of that original encounter with antigen.

Memory and naive T cells may be demonstrable in the laboratory. One surface molecule found on T cells is CD45. This molecule has been found to be altered when the T cell is activated by encounter with antigen (Figure 5.6). The original, or naive, T cell that has not yet encountered antigen is said to have the CD45RA molecule while the memory T cell has CD45RO. Unfortunately, recent data suggest that this distinction may not be entirely reliable. It is possible that cells can change from one CD45 format to another through events other than interaction with antigen.

Immune responses in specialized locations

The immune responses that have been described thus far are considered to take place in the very generalized environment of the circulation and extracellular spaces of the tissues (systemic immune system). Some specialized environments are home to responses that have some very distinctly different features. The immune responses that occur at mucosal surfaces are a good example. Most of the information we now have about such environments comes from work done on the immune systems of the gut and the respiratory tract. The skin presents a very effective

In the 1950s, it was unfortunate that a very eminent Nobel Prize winning British immunologists (Sir) Peter Medawar stated 'we shall come to regard the presence of lymphocytes in the thymus as an evolutionary accident of no very great significance'. Experimental work in the 1960s which investigated the effects of removing thymuses from newborn mice demonstrated the vital role of this organ in establishing the immune system that would last for the lifetime of the animal. Even this work did not refocus understanding because researchers were unable to detect antibody production in thymuses, and antibodies were seen as the defining feature of immune responses. The application of molecular biology techniques during the 1980s to discovering the nature and function of TCR has, at last, allowed us to move to our current position.

barrier between self and non-self but both natural and acquired immune responses in the inner layers of the skin have some very special features.

The gut and other mucosal surfaces

The immunocompetent cells present at mucosal surfaces are located in dispersed clumps of lymphoid tissue, termed **mucosa-associated lymphoid tissue (MALT)**. The importance of understanding the immune response associated with MALT is shown by the fact that the body's external surface, the skin, provides only some $2\,m^2$ across which potential pathogens may invade the body while the inner surfaces (gut, respiratory tract, etc.) present approximately $400\,m^2$. In the systemic immune system, when a T cell encounters foreign material, a vigorous response is initiated that ends only when the foreign material has been eliminated. Every day mucosae are exposed to a tremendous array of foreign matter. Within the gut, most of this is beneficial, i.e. foodstuffs, while other components are potentially hazardous, e.g. food-borne microorganisms. A response against all foreign material would be inappropriate. Current thinking is that foreign material that crosses the gut wall in high doses will induce a state of non-responsiveness, i.e. tolerance, termed **oral tolerance**, while that encountered in low doses will initiate protective responses (Figure 5.7). The tolerance is not confined to the local environment of the gut but can also occur systemically through lymphocyte re-circulation. In particular, there appears to be efficient transport of cells and molecules between the various locations of MALT. The immune cell types that are associated with MALT differ from those in the circulation. The lymphocytes, termed **intraepithelial lymphocytes (IEL)** are predominantly T cells bearing $\gamma\delta$ TCR (most circulating T cells have $\alpha\beta$ TCR). Specialized APCs are also present. These are the **M cells** that are found amongst the epithelial cells.

The immune response of mucosal surfaces also differs from that of the rest of the body in that its predominant antibody type is IgA. (IgG and IgM predominate elsewhere). This is thought to be because only IgA can be transported across epithelial cells to the lumen. The production of IgA does not only involve antibody-secreting plasma cells. The **secretory piece** that surrounds IgA (Chapter 4) is produced by the epithelial cells which the IgA must traverse on the journey from lymphoid tissue to the mucosal surface (Figure 5.8). The secretory piece is a member of the Ig gene superfamily (Chapter 4) but it is extensively glycosylated. Its gene locus is within the Class III region of the MHC. It is expressed as a cell surface molecule on the basal surface of mucosal epithelial cells but it then attaches to IgA and is secreted into the mucosal surface in that position. The function of the secretory piece is to provide a

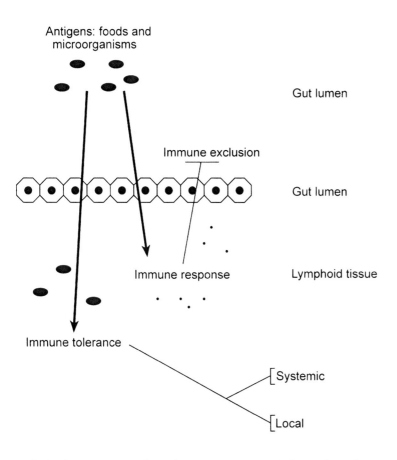

Antigens: foods and
microorganisms

Gut lumen

Immune exclusion

Gut lumen

Immune response

Lymphoid tissue

Immune tolerance

Systemic

Local

Figure 5.7 *Foreign material that crosses the gut wall in high doses will induce a state of non-responsiveness, i.e. tolerance, while that encounterd in low doses will initiate protective responses*

carbohydrate outer surface that can protect IgA from degradation by the proteolytic enzymes that share its mucosal environment.

The skin is comprised of a series of tissue layers at various depths from the surface (Figure 5.9). Most of the immune cell populations occur in the dermis with a few cells in the epidermis. Specialized APCs called **epidermal Langerhans cells** can migrate to the dermis, and from there to lymph nodes, to present antigen to T cells. Once in the lymph nodes the Langerhans cells are known as **dendritic cells**. Lymphocytes and other cell types present in the skin, e.g. **keratinocytes**, are rich sources of cytokines that are capable of

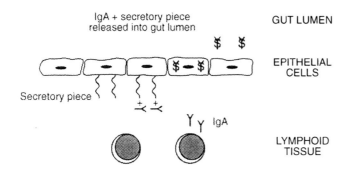

IgA + secretory piece
released into gut lumen

GUT LUMEN

EPITHELIAL
CELLS

Secretory piece

IgA

LYMPHOID
TISSUE

Figure 5.8 *IgA is produced in lymphoid tissue in the gut wall. To reach the gut lumen it must traverse epithelial cells that line the gut. During this traverse each IgA molecule acquires a secretory piece*

Figure 5.9 *The skin consists of a series of tissue layers. Antigen presentation to lymphocytes occurs predominantly in the dermis*

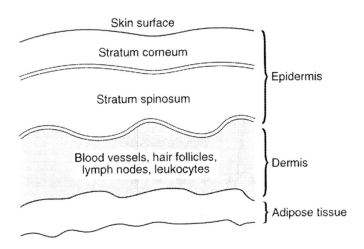

regulating local immune responses. Immune responses that are stimulated in the skin tend to be regarded as hypersensitivity responses, both cell-mediated **delayed-type hypersensitivity (DTH)** and antibody (IgE)-mediated **immediate hypersensitivity**. Both of these conditions are considered in detail in Chapter 7.

Interactions between the immune system, the nervous system and the endocrine system

The field concentrating on studies of interactions between the immune system and neuroendocrine organs (including, for example, brain, pituitary, thyroid, parathyroid, pancreas, adrenal glands, testes, ovary) has a number of names, including **psychoneuroimmunology** and **neuroimmunoendocrinology**.

Communication between these systems is suggested by several observations. Physical or emotional stress and psychiatric illness activate the endocrine system and can compromise immunological functions. The profound effect of stress on immune responses can, in turn, elicit marked physiological and chemical changes in the brain.

Direct modulation of the immune system by neuroendocrine influences can also be inferred from the innervation of immune organs such as spleen, thymus, and lymph nodes by sympathetic and sensory neurons. A neural supply to the immune system allows for local delivery of neuropeptides and other neuromediators at high concentrations, which can then act on receptors expressed on immune cells. The reciprocal entry of immune cells into the nervous system has also been observed. Monocytes, macrophages and T cells are able to cross the blood–brain barrier. Macrophages can persist for very long intervals as resident microglia of the brain and constitute approximately 10% of the total glial cell population. Activated T cells are retained for days if they react specifically with central nervous system antigens. A variety of stimuli have been shown to induce expression of MHC antigens on astrocytes, microglia and oligodendrocytes, which then can function to present antigens and to become targets for CTLs. Functionally significant concentrations of some neuropeptides are also found at sites of immune and inflammatory reactions.

A direct participation of the nervous system in immune functions is indicated by a number of observations. Destruction of the hypothalamus has been shown, for example, to reduce the number of large granular lymphocytes (LGL), the activity of NK cells, the ratio of $CD4^+/CD8^+$ T cells, and the level of circulating B cells. Firing rates of hypothalamic neurons have been shown to be altered during immune responses. Hypophysectomy is also known to cause an impairment of antibody and cell-mediated immunity, which can be corrected by treatment with neuromodulatory mediators such as prolactin, or growth hormone.

Many different classes of molecules, including cytokines and neurotransmitters, are involved in the amplification, coordination, and regulation of communication pathways within the neuroimmune system. It appears that these substances can act on neuroendocrine target cells in addition to regulating immune responses. It should be remembered that most, if not all, endocrine glands contain a high number of lymphocytes. For example, these cells can make up to 20% of the total cell number in the case of the adrenal gland. Moreover, many classical cytokines of the immune system have been shown to be produced by a variety of brain cells, including neurons and glial cells.

Neurohormonal involvement in immune reactions has been known for some time, in particular through the immunosuppressive effects of glucocorticoid hormones. Production from the adrenal gland of cortisol in humans is stimulated by ACTH, one of the many interactions that comprise the physiologically important regulatory entity known as the hypothalamic–pituitary–adrenocortical axis (HPA) or stress axis, which integrates functions of the hypothalamus, the pituitary and the adrenal glands. Recent evidence indicates that the immune system may also be a component of this regulatory group.

Other neuromodulators released from the neuronal systems and influencing cells of the immune system include, for example, β-endorphin, follicle-stimulating hormone (FSH), angiotensin, growth hormone, luteinizing hormone, prolactin, somatostatin, SP (substance P) and related tachykinins, thymic hormones, thyrotrophin, vasopressin, vasoactive intestinal peptide (VIP), and many other small oligopeptides, neurotransmitters, and non-protein molecules. Many of these factors have been shown to be released also by activated cells of the immune system. Immune cells have been shown to produce authentic neuromodulatory molecules identical to those produced by brain and nerve cells and to express functional receptors for those molecules. Precisely how these factors can modulate immunity and/or neuronal processes (cell growth, survival and differentiation) remains to be determined.

In addition to classical neuromodulatory factors, cytokines including, for example, IL-1, IL-2, IL-6, TNF-α and IFN also have potent neuroendocrine activities. Neuroimmunoendocrine factors thus are components of a complex signalling system that helps to maintain homeostasis by allowing cross-talk between the systems.

It is possible that the immune system possesses sensory functions with leukocytes identifying stimuli/stressor signals that are not recognizable by the nervous system. Cytokine receptors on cells of the immune and nervous system seem to play a sensory and regulatory role enabling the brain to monitor the progress of immune responses. The brain may be able also to modulate immune responses, for example, by using its neuroimmunomodulatory factors to alter the functional capacities of immune cells.

Many of these observations may help to clarify phenomena that have long been described but for which physiological evidence was lacking. The complexity of the system suggests that there will be no single unifying factor in nervous, endocrine and immune system interactions. Eventually, however, elucidation of the mechanisms underlying communication systems within the body may help to integrate fields as diverse as psychology, pathology and physiology.

Suggested further reading

Brandtzaeg, P., Baekkevold, E.S., Farstad, I.N., Jahnsen, F.L., Johansen, F-E, Nielsen, E.M. and Yamanaka, T. (1999) Regional specialization in the mucosal immune system: what happens in the microcompartments? *Immunology Today* 20, 141–151.

Cleland, J.L. (1999) Single-administration vaccines: controlled-release technology to mimic repeated immunizations. *Trends in Biotechnology* 17, 25–29.

Jepson, M.A. and Clark, M.A. (1999) Studying M cells and their role in infection. *Trends in Microbiology* 6, 359–365.

Paul, W.E. and Seder, R.A. (1994) Lymphocyte responses and cytokines. *Cell* 76, 241–251.

Peters, J.H., Gieseler, R., Thiele, B. and Steinbach, F. (1996) Dendritic cells: from ontogenic orphans to myelomonocytic descendants. *Immunology Today* 17, 273–278.

Rajewsky, K. (1998) Burnet's unhappy hybrid. *Nature* 394, 624–625.

Wilckens, T. and DeRijk, R. (1997) Glucocorticoids and immune function: unknown dimensions and new frontiers. *Immunology Today* 18, 418–424.

Strobel, S. and Mowat, A.McI. (1998) Immune responses to dietary antigens: oral tolerance. *Immunology Today* 19, 173–181.

Zinkernagel, R.M., Bachmann, M.F., Kundig, T.M., Oehen, S., Pirchet, H. and Hengartner, H. (1996) On immunological memory. *Annual Review of Immunology* **14**, 333–367.

Self-assessment questions

1. List two ways in which the predominant antibodies of a secondary immune response differ from those in the primary response.
2. Name one type of microorganism that will induce CTL production.
3. Name one type of microorganism that will induce IgA production and state its most likely route of entry into the body.
4. In a secondary response the cytokines IL-2 and IFN-γ are produced. What is the nature of the responding T cells?
5. List three immunological mechanisms that are used to combat viral infections.
6. Explain why it is not necessary for B cells to undergo selection following random re-arrangement of their antigen receptors in the way that T cells do.
7. List 10 events that occur following TCR binding to MHC + antigen but before IgM secretion.
8. What are T cell co-stimulators?
9. Oral tolerance is currently an experimental clinical technique by which autoimmune responses in diseases such as multiple sclerosis may be down-regulated. Give the scientific rationale for this approach.
10. If an antigen enters the body by crossing the skin, where is the immune response most likely to take place?

Key Concepts and Facts

Characteristics of Acquired Immune Responses
- Acquired immune responses display specificity and memory.

- If CD8$^+$ T cells are stimulated with MHC Class I + antigen a cell-mediated response occurs. If CD4$^+$ T cells are stimulated with MHC Class II + antigen an antibody-mediated response occurs.

- Secondary immune responses are swifter and more effective than primary responses.

Cell-mediated Responses
- The CD8$^+$ T cells proliferate and differentiate to become cytotoxic T cells (CTL).

- The CTL kill virally infected or tumour target cells.

- Killing by CTLs involves pore-forming perforins and lymphotoxin (LT, TNF-β).

Antibody-mediated Responses
- The CD4$^+$ T cells proliferate and activate antigen-specific B cells.

- The B cells proliferate and differentiate to become antibody-secreting plasma cells.

- Antibodies interact with target cells, molecules, bacteria, fungi, yeasts or extracellular virus particles.

- Antibodies activate complement and the opsonized targets are phagocytosed.

Immune Responses at Specialized Sites
- Immune responses at mucosal surfaces involve IgA and tolerance is more readily established than in the circulation.

- Immune responses occur in the dermis of the skin and in adjacent lymph nodes.

- A complex communications network exists between the immune, nervous and endocrine systems.

Chapter 6
Infection and immunity

Learning objectives

After studying this chapter you should confidently be able to:

Describe the type of immune response likely to be elicited by a particular infectious microorganism.

Discuss the possible pathological consequences of immune and inflammatory responses against microorganisms.

Discuss the mechanisms used by microorganisms to avoid destruction by immune responses.

Describe the strategy behind the development of successful vaccines and discuss current new approaches.

Infectious diseases may be considered to occur because of the inability of host immune responses to eliminate **pathogenic (i.e. disease-causing)** infectious microorganisms. Some individuals mount very effective immune responses to infection, while others respond poorly or not at all.

The level of response is determined by several factors including:

- The nature of the infecting microorganism.
- The extent of infection.
- Factors related to the efficacy of the host immune response, e.g. MHC haplotype, T cell numbers, T cell function.
- Other genetic factors that contribute to the outcome of the disease.
- Other host factors such as the presence of other infections that may cause immunosuppression (e.g. HIV), the use of immuno-suppressive drugs (e.g. anti-rejection drugs) and the presence of immunodeficiency disorders (Chapter 9).

Microorganisms that establish infections only in individuals with breaks in their physical defences, e.g. wounds, or compromised (suppressed) immune systems are known as **opportunistic pathogens.**

In some infectious diseases the extent of host immune reactivity may be correlated with MHC specificities, i.e. some alleles of MHC genes present immunogenic (immunostimulatory) antigens more effectively than do other alleles. Molecular analysis of allelic forms of MHC molecules is now yielding more information on this MHC–disease relationship. While it is now possible to determine the sequence of each MHC allele, a major impediment exists in trying to link this sequence with function in the presentation of specific microbial antigens. The problem is that so few of the important microbial antigens have yet been identified. In the future the analysis of MHC associations with infectious diseases should allowed precise definition of susceptibility and protective alleles in populations of different ethnic origins and, ultimately, in individuals. Such information could eventually be used to define populations, or individuals, who may be at greater risk from particular infections.

Currently, we can distinguish readily the types of immune mechanisms that are used to combat the various different types of infectious microorganisms. Very frequently, people with deficiencies in particular components of the immune system have an increased susceptibility to infection with defined microorganisms (Chapter 9). Effective protection against infectious diseases requires a combination of both natural and acquired immune responses.

Responses to bacteria

The body's many physical and chemical barriers, and the presence of normal bacterial flora on the skin and internal mucosal surfaces, effectively limit the ability of bacteria to invade the body (Chapter 2). Those which do gain entry are rapidly targeted by natural immunity. The acquired response to bacteria is predominantly antibody-mediated. Antibody can neutralize the toxins produced by several pathogenic bacteria, for example, diphtheria or cholera toxins. It also activates complement which is particularly effective against Gram-negative bacteria (Figure 6.1). IgA in the lumen of

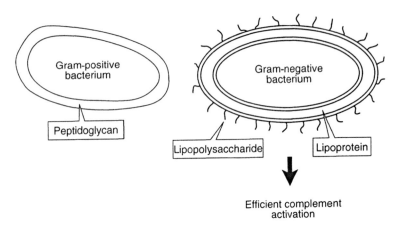

Figure 6.1 *Antibody can neutralize the toxins produced by several pathogenic bacteria, e.g. diphtheria toxin. It also activates complement which is particularly effective against Gram-negative bacteria*

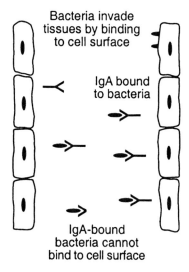

Bacteria invade
tissues by binding
to cell surface

IgA bound
to bacteria

IgA-bound
bacteria cannot
bind to cell surface

GUT LUMEN   EPITHELIAL
LAYER

Figure 6.2 *IgA in the lumen of the gut and other hollow organs with mucosal surfaces, i.e. respiratory tract and genito-urinary tracts, decreases pathogen invasion into tissues. The IgA can bind to microorganisms, so inhibiting their attachment to the gut wall*

the gut and other hollow organs with mucosal surfaces, i.e. respiratory tract and genito–urinary tracts, is important in preventing microorganisms from binding to the gut wall and so gaining access to tissues (Figure 6.2). IgA differs from other antibody isotypes in that it activates complement via the **alternate pathway**.

Most bacteria are killed by phagocytes but some can escape these responses. These include *Mycobacterium leprae* and *Mycobacterium tuberculosis* which cause the diseases of leprosy and tuberculosis, respectively. These are intracellular bacteria, i.e. they live within host macrophages. The consequences of this inability of phagocytes to kill and eliminate phagocytosed microorganisms are significant:

- The natural immune response (acute inflammation) cannot be terminated because the antigen cannot be removed from the body. This leads to the pathological condition known as **chronic inflammation, also termed Type IV hypersensitivity** (Chapter 7).

- The microorganisms may live in a dormant state within the phagocytes but may be allowed to become activated, for example through immune suppression due to AIDS or malnutrition. The mycobacteria then replicate leading to a re-emergence of the disease.

When host macrophages are stimulated by the cytokine interferon γ (IFN-γ) from CD4$^+$ Th1 cells (Chapter 5) the mycobacteria are likely to be killed.

Contrary to how it may sometimes appear, it is not advantageous to an infectious microorganism to kill its host. When the host is dead, the microorganism no longer has a place to live and replicate. Some of the most successful pathogens are those that have evolved to be able to live together with the host over long periods of time. This is known as chronic infection.

Genetic factors may control host responses to *Mycobacterium tuberculosis*. Population studies have determined an association between pulmonary tuberculosis (TB) and MHC specificities. The MHC allele HLA-DR2 is associated with the development of both TB and leprosy. When the sequence of Class II alleles in patients with pulmonary TB and drug-resistant TB is available, it may be possible to identify an amino acid residue(s) critical for the binding of *M. tuberculosis*-derived pathogenic peptide(s).

MHC alleles also modulate the immune response that determines the form of leprosy that develops in each patient. It may be:

- lepromatous leprosy (LL), in patients who are weakly responsive to the antigens of *M. leprae*;
- tuberculoid leprosy (TT), in patients who exhibit a good cell-mediated immune response, i.e. CD4$^+$ Th1 cells predominate;
- intermediate features.

An increased frequency of HLA-DR2 and HLA-DQ1 has been seen in LL patients while increased HLA-DR3 in TT patients has been reported. These antigens can be further subdivided into alleles defined by their amino acid sequence. A single amino acid substitution may give rise to alleles with different immunological properties that might modulate the immune response and determine the form of leprosy that develops in each patient.

Not all damage to the host that is associated with infectious diseases is actually caused directly by the infecting microorganisms. Immune responses to bacterial infections may be potentially lethal to the host in the condition known variously as **septicaemia; bacteraemia; sepsis; septic shock or Type V hypersensitivity** (Chapter 7). The symptoms of septic shock are:

- excessively high and prolonged fever;
- diffuse intravascular coagulation (i.e. blood clotting within many vessels throughout the body);
- hypotension;
- circulatory collapse;
- haemorrhagic necrosis.

The development of a septicaemia is frequently recognized only in a relatively late stage by the drop in blood pressure. The patient dies from multi-organ failure. Management of the shock-specific symptoms is still one of the most challenging problems faced by clinicians. The principal components of immune responses that induce septic shock appear to be the pro-inflammatory cytokines (IL-1, IL-6 and TNF-α, Chapter 3).

The existence of the profound and rapid cytokine-mediated response known as septic shock may, in fact, represent a very important evolutionary development. Within a population, when one person acquires an infectious disease, that disease can spread to many others with whom the initial patient comes into contact. The greater the number of contacts, the greater is the risk to the population. The very swift death of a person with a serious infectious disease will restrict significantly the spread of the infection.

Responses to fungi and yeasts

The precise mechanisms involved in fungal immunity are poorly defined. There may be some neutrophil activity and T cells secrete cytokines to activate macrophages which kill the fungi. Antibody-mediated immune responses may also occur. Infections with the yeast *Candida albicans* are common in immunosuppressed patients therefore acquired responses normally keep this infection in check. Invasive fungal infections may also occur following organ transplantation. Most infections occur within the first month after transplantation and are usually caused by *Candida* organisms.

The clinical features of invasive fungal infections in immunocompromised patients may include fever and leukocytosis (i.e. massively increased numbers of leukocytes in the circulation), but the most common are disturbances in the function of the involved organ. Intravascular catheters are another important site of *Candida* infections. Organisms generally gain access from colonized skin surfaces and adhere to the intravascular device. Early diagnosis of invasive fungal infections in patients is a desirable but elusive goal. Diagnosis is based primarily on clinical signs and 'suspicion', because blood cultures are often negative. Unfortunately, because of the lack of specific signs and symptoms, treatment is often delayed. Treatment itself, especially in the case of patients receiving the immunosuppressive drug **cyclosporin** (the most common immunosuppressant currently used) may be problematic. This is because cyclosporin is nephrotoxic and is metabolized by the hepatic cytochrome P450 enzyme system. Many antifungals inhibit cytochrome P450 enzymes so their co-administration with cyclosporin will result in increased cyclosporin levels and will almost certainly contribute to nephrotoxicity. Also, resistance to antifungal drugs is a growing problem.

Responses to parasites

Parasitic infections are a major problem especially in tropical countries where the effects may be exacerbated by malnutrition. A single parasite may also present many different targets because of existing in several different forms during a complex life-cycle. Some of the developmental forms of parasites may be extracellular while others are intracellular. **Malaria** is one of the most widespread of diseases, killing up to 2 million people annually. Where parasitic worms are endemic, stunted growth and mental retardation in children may occur. Both antibody and cell-mediated responses may be stimulated depending upon the particular infecting organism. In general terms, organisms which invade the bloodstream, e.g. *Plasmodium falciparum* (causes malaria), *Trypanosoma spp.* (cause trypanosomiasis), induce antibody production while those which live in tissues are associated with cell-mediated responses.

Helminthic (worm) infections involve elevated IgE levels and increased recruitment of eosinophils.

Some protozoan parasites may escape from killing by macrophages and live within those cells following phagocytosis. *Toxoplasma gondii*, *Trypanosoma cruzi* and *Leishmania spp.* are examples of these protozoans. As with intracellular bacteria, IFN-γ from T cells is essential to activate the macrophages and so overcome the infection. The possession of genes for certain MHC proteins appears to favour effective anti-parasite responses accounting, in part, for different racial susceptibilities. Many parasitic infections are not cleared but enter a chronic phase which may extend over many years. The immune/inflammatory response continues throughout this time causing damage to the host.

Infection with *T. gondii* induces a humoral immune response with production of specific IgG, IgM, IgA and IgE. Specific antibody, combined with complement, lyses extracellular parasites at the tachyzoite stage. Tachyzoites coated with antibody can also passively enter phagocytes via Fc receptors. CD4$^+$ Th1-cell function appears to be important in the defence against infection, for example, as a source of the IFN-γ that activates macrophages for anti-toxoplasma activity. These mechanisms account for the limited course of the infection in the normal, acutely infected host. They also contribute to containment of the chronic form of infection when the organism may persist in the form of latent tissue cysts. In patients with severe defects in cell-mediated immunity, the process of containment of tissue cysts is compromised. Groups of people at increased risk include those immunosuppressed following transplants, patients with AIDS or cancer, or patients taking long-term corticosteroids. The onset of the immune suppression can be associated with the **reactivation of latent infection**. Encephalitis (inflammation of the brain) is the most common manifestation of toxoplasmosis seen in both AIDS and non-AIDS immunocompromised hosts.

Chagas' disease, caused by the protozoan parasite *Trypanosoma cruzi*, is an important cause of morbidity in many countries in Latin America. The important modes of transmission are by the bite of the reduviid bug and blood transfusion. Parasite adherence to, and invasion of, host cells is a complex process involving complement and a series of degradative enzymes. Two clinical forms of the disease are recognized: acute and chronic. During the acute stage pathological damage is related to the presence of the parasite whereas, in the chronic stage, few parasites are found. In recent years the roles of TNF-α, IFN-γ and the interleukins in the pathogenesis of this infection have been reported. The common symptoms are chronic cardiac arrhythmias and thromboemboli (blood clots in the lungs). The gastrointestinal tract is another important target. Exacerbations of *T. cruzi* infection have been reported for patients receiving immunosuppressive therapy and for those with AIDS.

Table 6.1 *Each type of hypersensitivity reaction (Chapter 7) may be stimulated by particular infectious microorganisms*

Hypersensitivity	Infectious organism
Type I	Ascaris (a worm)
Type II	Trypanosoma cruzi
Type III	Plasmodium falciparum (causes malaria)
Type IV	Eggs of Schistosoma (a worm), Leishmania
Type V	Plasmodium falciparum

MHC association with parasitic infections

Malaria-exposed and unexposed populations show differences in the frequencies of MHC Class I genes at the A and B loci. It may be hypothesized that the MHC complex protects populations in disease endemic areas who are exposed to malaria parasites. The association between the MHC Class I antigen HLA-B53 and protection from severe malaria has already been established. The pin-pointing of prevalent MHC alleles within an at-risk population may assist in the development of specific vaccines that would be presented efficiently and so induce effective immune responses. Parasites may act as the stimuli for hypersensitivity reactions (Chapter 7). Some examples are shown in Table 6.1.

Responses to viruses

The earliest responses to viruses involve NK cells, IFN-α and IFN-β. The cytokines induce an **antiviral state** in which adjacent cells are resistant to infection. Some viruses decrease cellular expression of MHC Class I antigens, thereby precipitating attack by NK cells. Natural killer cells are further stimulated by IFN-γ. When viral antigens are presented in association with Class I MHC, cytotoxic T cell responses can be targeted against the virally infected cells.

The most significant effectors in the acquired response are cytotoxic CD8$^+$ T cells although CD4$^+$ cells also contribute by releasing cytokines to activate macrophages and by producing antibodies. Some antibodies, with complement, may neutralize viruses. Phagocytes also engulf extracellular virus particles. This phenomenon would contribute to the large numbers of HIV particles found within macrophages in infected patients. Macrophages, unlike T cells, are not killed but act as reservoirs of HIV even when circulating virus is undetectable.

The types of responses directed against some tumours and to cells in mis-matched transplants or transfusions are thought to be the same as those directed against viruses.

The many alleles of MHC genes, encoding many allotypes of MHC antigens, each of which binds to and presents a slightly different epitope, can be a real advantage to a population. Different alleles in different people would allow each to respond more effectively to a particular set of infectious microorganisms. This means that when one pathogenic microorganism enters the population some people may succumb to the infection while others survive, i.e. those who mounted the best response would survive. The extreme variability of MHC antigens allows that, for any microorganism, there should always be somebody in the group who can survive an epidemic. An isolated, in-bred, population will display less variability in MHC therefore, while everybody may mount effective responses against some microorganisms, they may be at greater risk of complete elimination if faced with some other infectious agents.

MHC association with viral infections

There is now just a little information about associations between MHC alleles and anti-viral immune responses. Transmission of HIV-1 from an infected woman to her offspring during gestation and delivery is known to be influenced by the infant's MHC Class II DRB1 alleles.

An estimated 250 million people throughout the world are chronically infected with hepatitis B virus, the primary cause of chronic hepatitis, cirrhosis and hepatocellular carcinoma in disease-endemic regions. Because MHC Class I antigens contain viral peptides, they may be important targets for immune mediated destruction of hepatocytes by $CD8^+$ CTLs in hepatitis B virus infection. Prognosis may be quite different among patients infected with hepatitis C virus: a chronic liver disease occurs in half the patients, while the other half exhibits no histological signs of progression of liver damage. The host immune responses may play an important role in such different outcomes. The level of serum MHC Class I antigens increases markedly during the course of many viral infections and, during HIV-1 infection, the level of serum MHC Class I antigens correlates with disease stage.

Subverting the immune response – microbial evasion strategies

The survival needs of microorganisms that cause infectious diseases in humans have caused them to develop methods to protect themselves against complete elimination by immune responses. The evasion strategies used are many and varied. They include both mechanisms to reduce the effectiveness of responses and to allow the microorganisms to achieve a safe haven in the face of an intact response.

Microbial activities that suppress immune responses include:

1. **Production of enzymes that degrade proteins of the immune response**

   Bacteria

   - Streptococcal proteases can lyse complement factors.
   - Gonococci and meningococci secrete proteases that degrade IgA.

   Parasites

   - *Leishmania* can produce a molecule similar to decay accelerating factor that degrades complement.
   - Roundworms secrete proteases that degrade antibodies.

   Viruses

   - Herpes simplex virus produces proteins that degrade complement factors.

2. Secretion of toxins to kill immune cells or inhibit their functions

Bacteria

- Streptolysin from streptococci kills neutrophils and inhibits neutrophil chemotaxis.
- Mycobacteria prevent phagosome–lysosome fusion in macrophages and *shigella* may escape from phagosomes.
- Staphylococcal or streptococcal protein A and protein G block the Fc ends of antibodies so that they cannot bind to Fc receptors.
- Pneumococci and meningococci form a polysaccharide capsule that decreases adherence to phagocytes and may inactivate bound complement factors.
- Staphylococci form an outer coat of host fibrin that inactivates complement.

Fungi

- *Cryptococcus* can degrade the reactive oxygen species produced during the oxidative burst of phagocytes.

Parasites

- Toxoplasma inhibits phagosome–lysosome fusion. Leishmania prevents cytokine production by T cells.

Viruses

- Adenoviruses and Epstein Barr Virus (EBV) can disrupt the anti-viral state induced by IFN.
- EBV can produce a cytokine-like molecule that mimics IL-10 (IL-10 down-regulates inflammatory responses).
- Herpes viruses and adenoviruses can bind to MHC antigens to down-regulate their functions.

3. Direct infection of immune cells

Viruses

- T-cell infection and destruction by HIV and B cell infection by EBV.

Ways in which microorganisms can 'hide' from the immune response include:

1. Antigenic variation

Bacteria

- Gonococci, streptococci and *Escherichia coli* vary the structure of outer surface proteins so they develop a vast number of antigenically different strains. On each occasion that a person is infected with an organism it is treated as being a 'new' antigen and only primary responses can be mounted.

Parasites

- The complex lifecycle of many parasites means that one organism can exist in several antigenically different stages. Further, the antigens expressed at any one stage may vary from organism to organism, e.g. in trypanosomes.

Viruses

- HIV, influenza virus and rhinovirus (causes the common cold) change their surface antigens rapidly giving rise to many new strains and preventing effective immunological memory. Constant small changes in antigen occur. However, sometimes, there are larger antigenic shifts that can give rise to global epidemics, called pandemics, for example, the influenza pandemics of 1918 (where more people were killed than in both world wars together), 1957 and 1968.

2. **Antigen masking**

Parasites

- The worm *Shistosoma mansoni* coats itself with host molecules, e.g. MHC antigens, so that it is not recognized as being foreign.

3. **Shedding of surface antigens**

Parasites

- *Leishmania* and *Plasmodium* may shed large quantities of surface antigen that bind to antibodies and so block their interactions with the organism

4. **Replication inside host cells**

Bacteria

- Intracellular bacteria, e.g. Mycobacteria, replicate in phagosomes of macrophages.

Parasites

- *Plasmodium falciparum* (which causes malaria) replicates in erythrocytes.
- *Leishmania* and *Toxoplasma* replicate in phagosomes of macrophages while *T. Cruzi* replicates in the cytosol.
- Worms such as *Trinchinella* hide inside cysts that are resistant to immune killing.

5. **Latency (microorganisms can infect host cells and remain dormant there for many years).**

Bacteria

- Intracellular bacteria such as mycobacteria may reside for may years within macrophages only re-commencing replication if the immune system is suppressed.

Viruses

- Once the HIV genome is incorporated into a host cell, e.g. a T cell, it may remain dormant for up to at least 15 years. The factors that cause latency to end and replication to begin are not well understood.

- Some herpes viruses survive within the genomes of nerve cells.

Vaccines

The observation that a person who recovered from an infectious disease would subsequently be immune to the same disease was made many times, over many centuries. Indeed the deliberate exposure of children and adults to infection in order to assure later protection was practised in many societies across the world. In May 1796 Edward Jenner, a medical practitioner in Gloucestershire, England, inoculated an 8-year-old boy with matter taken from a milkmaid's cowpox pustule. This brave step had been inspired by the observation that people who contracted the mild infection called cowpox did not get smallpox, then a much feared, often fatal disease. In July of the same year the boy was inoculated with smallpox and remained healthy. Following publication of his findings, Jenner's **vaccination** technique was widely adopted. Once Jenner found that an effective vaccine could be made from dried lymph taken from the smallpox pustules, he was able to send vaccine to colleagues many miles away and so increase the frequency of vaccination.

Jenner was the first to take a rational, scientific approach to the manipulation of human immune responses. His approach was to develop **active immunity**, i.e. the patient's own immune system responded to the potential pathogen to bring about protective immunity. **Passive immunization**, on the other hand, involves the administration of pre-formed antibodies (in antiserum) to a patient who has been exposed, or is at risk of exposure to, an infectious pathogen. The antiserum must initially be made in another host, frequently in horses. Early attempts to use horse antisera encountered problems known as 'serum sickness'. This was caused by the fact that the horse antibodies are regarded by the patient's immune system as being foreign. A vigorous immune response was mounted against the horse antiserum causing a build-up of **immune complexes**, i.e. amalgamations of antigen and antibody, within the patient's circulation. This response is detailed in Chapter 7 under the heading of **Type III Hypersensitivity**. A further drawback is that passive immunization does not allow the development of specific memory. The antibodies that are given to a person are gradually removed from the circulation so must be re-administered if needed in the future. Passive immunization is now carried out only in emergency situations. These include cases where the patient has been exposed to something so toxic that they would die before an immune response was mounted, e.g. tetanus toxin or snakebite

The practice of vaccination in western Europe had royal beginnings. Lady Mary Wortley Montagu, wife of the (then) British ambassador to Turkey learned of the practice of inoculation and, in Istanbul in the early years of the eighteenth century, had her 6-year-old son vaccinated against smallpox. She returned to England in 1718 and campaigned in support of the technique. The Prince of Wales, later King George I, ordered that some condemned criminals should be inoculated. When these people survived, two young princesses were also treated. This started something of a 'fashion' for inoculation, however it was only practised infrequently and was not examined seriously until Edward Jenner's day.

'Everybody in the public health field knows that when you reach the point where you can begin to inoculate an agent into millions of children, your problems have only just begun.' This quote is from Albert Sabin who developed the Sabin oral vaccine for poliomyelitis.

Note: The words inoculation, vaccination and immunization tend to be used interchangeably.

venom, or in the case of pregnant women who cannot be exposed to many of the current vaccines because of the risk to the foetus.

Active immunization is, normally, only carried out on healthy people. The practice of giving a medicine to a healthy child or adult would appear to run contrary to most people's concept of healthcare. Thus the efficacy and potential benefit of immunization must always be balanced carefully against the potential risk to the individual. A number of different types of vaccines have been developed to cope with a wide range of diseases. The types of vaccine currently used are:

- **Attenuated vaccines and inactivated vaccines.** Attenuated (weakened) bacteria or viruses have been manipulated *in vitro* so that they can induce only a very mild infection, i.e. they are weakly virulent. The risk attached is that a mutation may occur to restore virulence. A safeguard against this is either the removal of the virulence genes or the inactivation (killing) of the organism so that it cannot replicate *in vivo*. Attenuated vaccines are the more potent as the response that is induced resembles the natural response. Killed viruses usually generate only antibody-mediated immunity and, because the organisms in the vaccine cannot replicate, they usually have to be repeated (booster injections) to maintain the required level of immunity. A person who is immune suppressed cannot be given an attenuated vaccine because even a mild infection might prove lethal.

- **Purified subunit vaccines.** These vaccines comprise only some of the antigens expressed by the intact microorganism. These are the immunodominant antigens so usually they are derived from the outer cell surface of the microorganism, e.g. bacterial polysaccharides or components of the viral surface antigens. In order to evoke a more powerful immune response, the purified subunit may be conjugated to a protein that will stimulate $CD4^+$ T cells and thus a powerful antibody-mediated response. These are known as **conjugate vaccines.**

- **Toxoids.** A number of microorganisms cause disease by producing toxins. The organisms themselves, in the absence of toxin, are not pathogenic. Toxoids are inactivated toxins that induce immunity to toxin, not to the microorganism.

Most vaccine preparations contain an **adjuvant.** Adjuvants boost the immune responses against the antigen(s) in the vaccine. Alum is a commonly used adjuvant for human vaccines.

Measles vaccine

For most of the twentieth century measles epidemics regularly struck large numbers of children. The aftermath of measles can include serious diseases or blindness, thought to be due to the immune suppression following the infection. In the 1940s the virus was killing several hundred children each year in the UK. The first measles vaccines were introduced in 1968 and the number of cases declined rapidly.

In 1988 the UK government introduced the combined measles, mumps and rubella (MMR) triple vaccine. The proportion of 2-year-olds immunized rose to more than 90%. The vaccine contains live attenuated virus and is offered for babies with a booster shot at about 4 years of age. Measles, once a common cause of blindness and brain damage, has now been all but eradicated in westernized countries.

Polio vaccine

Inactivated polio vaccine (IPV) was used in the USA between 1955 and 1961. Since then the live attenuated vaccine, also known as the Salk or oral polio vaccine (OPV), has been the preferred vaccine because it is easier to administer and because it confers what is known as 'intestinal immunity' (i.e. IgA) in addition to stimulating the production of other antibodies. Because OPV contains live virus, however, reversion to virulence can cause a vaccinated child, the child's contacts or immunosuppressed individuals, to develop vaccine-associated paralytic poliomyelitis (VAPP).

There have been no cases of wild-type polio in the US since 1979, but the number of VAPP cases due to OPV reversion to virulence occurs at a rate of about 8–10 cases annually. IPV is not associated with a risk for VAPP. It has been used for more than 40 years in Western Europe, Scandinavia, and Canada. Because IPV and later, enhanced inactivated polio vaccine (eIPV), has been used in many Western European and Scandinavian countries, outbreaks of wild-type polio are practically non-existent in these countries. Notably, there have been very rare small outbreaks of wild-type polio in countries using IPV, in Sweden and the Netherlands, that were due to importation and subsequent transmission of wild virus within sections of the population that refused immunization.

Diphtheria–tetanus–pertussis (DTP) combination vaccines

In the mid-1970s reports of damage from whooping cough (pertussis) vaccine led to a nationwide scare and the establishment of a UK government compensation scheme. The proportion of children being immunized against whooping cough fell from more than 80% to about 30%. Within a few years, a series of epidemics had affected nearly 250 000 and resulted in dozens of deaths.

The combination DTP vaccine (diphtheria–tetanus toxoids–acellular pertussis) is now used for children aged 2, 4 and 6 months. Pharmaceutical companies are now testing new multivalent vaccines that will add in other vaccines against viruses such as *Haemophilus influenzae* type B (HiB, a conjugated vaccine of bacterial polysaccharide and protein), hepatitis B (HepB, an inactive viral vaccine), polio (eIPV) and chickenpox (*varicella-zoster*). It is hoped that safe, efficacious, multivalent vaccines will reduce the number of injections per visit to the Health Centre thus, potentially, increasing immunization rates and decreasing cost.

Varicella–Zoster Virus (chickenpox) vaccine

An interesting controversy in the USA surrounds the use of the varicella vaccine, a live attenuated virus, which has been on the market since May 1995. For a time parents and doctors alike hesitated to use the varicella vaccine because of the debate about whether a child might be better off getting chickenpox naturally.

The varicella vaccine has been used for about 10 years in Japan where studies there confirm that continued immunity has been established for at least that long. The increasing danger of group A streptococcus infection (the so-called 'flesh-eating bacteria') in children with chickenpox provides another reason for childhood immunization against chickenpox.

Pneumococcal vaccine

A number of pneumococcal conjugate (Pnc) vaccines have undergone safety and immunogenicity trials. Such a vaccine is recommended for use in adults over age 65 and people between the ages of 2 and 65 who might be immunocompromised or have other conditions, such as asplenia (lack of a spleen and, hence, some loss of immune function) or diabetes. This vaccine is effective against bacteraemia (bacteria in the bloodstream) and meningitis, but does not seem effective against otitis media (middle ear infection) or pneumonia without bacteraemia.

Hepatitis A vaccine

A vaccine for hepatitis A has been available for a number of years. Hepatitis A is primarily transmitted by person-to-person contact but infections from contaminated food and water also occur. Poor sanitation and crowding facilitate transmission. It is likely that hepatitis A immunization will become routine in the near future. Current developments in vaccine production use the techniques of molecular biology to create synthetic vaccines. These attempts promise to create effective vaccines without the risk of causing infection that accompanies vaccines based upon living, or once living, microorganisms. New approaches include:

- Production of **synthetic peptides** that mimic the epitopes that are presented by MHC antigens to induce immune responses.
- **Transfection** of a non-pathogenic virus, e.g. *Vaccinia* (the cause of cowpox), with genes for immunodominant antigens of

pathogens. The harmless *Vaccinia* will replicate thus increasing the dose of the foreign antigen and ensuring an effective response.

A current major goal of immunologists worldwide is the production of a vaccine against the human immunodeficiency virus (HIV). Research centres are using both 'traditional' and novel techniques to produce a safe and effective vaccine.

In the two centuries since Jenner's important discovery, public interest in safe and effective vaccination has not waned. Nonetheless, despite the availability and dependable quality of vaccines for childhood illnesses, it has been estimated that, in the USA, only 67% of children receive their vaccinations on time. Nonetheless, childhood remains the most opportune time during which infectious diseases may be controlled. Will the introduction of new vaccines prove a cost-effective way to improve our health or will it just complicate an already complex (and expensive) immunization schedule? Worldwide, the economic costs of immunization programmes frequently causes them to become political 'hot potatoes'. The poorer countries of the world often are those where infectious diseases have their greatest prevalence and where immunization programmes could show the most significant benefit. Malaria is an example of a disease that is endemic in developing countries that cannot afford large-scale vaccine development. There is little willingness on the part of major pharmaceutical companies to invest in vaccines when drugs to treat the illness continue to be profitable.

Many immunization programmes have been victims of the shortages created in the independent republics that emerged from the Soviet Union. Another critical problem facing immunization programmes is the reuse of disposable syringes or the use of improperly sterilized syringes and needles because of inadequate supplies. These practices can result in cross-infection with HIV, the hepatitis B virus, or other pathogens. In several countries new organizational structures must be established to deliver vaccinations to those at risk, especially children.

Suggested further reading

Brostoff, J., Scadding, G.K., Male, D. and Roitt, I.M. (1991) Clinical Immunology. London: Gower Medical Publishing.

Hill, A.V.S. (1998) The immunogenetics of human infectious diseases. *Annual Review of Immunology* **16**, 593–618.

Karlen, A. (1995) Plague's Progress. London: Victor Gollancz.

Shearer, G.M. and Clerici, M. (1997) Vaccine strategies: selective elicitation of cellular or humoral immunity? *Trends in Biotechnology* **15**, 106–109.

Self-assessment questions

1. List two factors that increase a person's chance of getting an opportunistic infection.
2. In the case of each of the infectious agents listed below, indicate whether cell-mediated immunity (CMI), antibody-mediated immunity (Ab) or both, would be more likely to be effective:
   (a) *Mycobacterium tuberculosis*
   (b) *Escherichia coli*
   (c) *Trypanosoma gondii*
3. Why are fungal infections difficult to treat in patients who have undergone organ transplantation?
4. What type of infection may be combated with raised IgE levels?
5. Why is it difficult for the immune system to eliminate intracellular bacteria?
6. Why are the anti-HIV antibodies that are produced early in the infection unable to clear the virus from the body?
7. Distinguish between the possible roles of the immune system in the diseases caused by hepatitis B and hepatitis C viruses.
8. How does the development of an outer coat of host fibrin help staphylococci to evade immune responses?
9. Give two possible disadvantages of passive immunization.
10. Why should it be safe for an immunosuppressed patient to receive a purified subunit vaccine but not an attenuated vaccine?

Key Concepts and Facts

Immune Responses to Bacteria
- Bacteria are effectively limited by the body's physical and chemical barriers and normal microbial flora.

- Extracellular bacteria are eliminated by cell-mediated immunity.

- Intracellular bacteria can evade phagocyte killing and persist. Activation of phagocytes with IFN-γ can increase their killing of intracellular organisms.

- Host damage following bacterial infections may be due to the strong cytokine-mediated immune responses that are initiated.

Immune Responses to Fungi and Yeasts
- Fungi and yeasts induce both cell-mediated and antibody-mediated immune responses.

Immune Responses to Parasites
- Both cell-mediated and antibody-mediated immune responses are activated.

- Differences in MHC alleles may allow some populations to respond to parasitic infections, for example malaria, better than others.

Immune Responses to Viruses
- Cell-mediated immunity involving CTLs and phagocytes is effective against viruses.

- The tissue damage associated with viral infection may be caused by the action of CTLs directed against virally infected cells.

Evasion of Host Immune Responses
- Many types of microorganism have evolved mechanisms to allow them to avoid destruction by the immune system.

- The principal evasion mechanisms involve disruption of immune responses and concealment of the organism from the cells and molecules of the immune system.

Vaccines
- The range of different vaccines now available includes live attenuated vaccines; killed vaccines; purified subunit vaccines; conjugate vaccines and toxoids.

- Active immunization aims to generate immunological memory and a full range of protective responses without risk to the person.

- Passive immunization involves administration of pre-formed antibodies and is used only in emergencies.

Chapter 7
Hypersensitivity

Learning objectives

After studying this chapter you should confidently be able to:

Describe the immunological mechanisms underlying five types of hypersensitivity responses.

Describe the principal causes and symptoms associated with hypersensitivity responses.

Discuss current approaches to the prevention or relief of hypersensitivity responses.

Hypersensitivity

A hypersensitivity reaction may be defined as:

an immune or inflammatory response that occurs in an exaggerated or inappropriate form, or in an inappropriate situation.

Thus normal effector mechanisms may passively damage host tissues. The response may be characteristic of an individual, i.e. it may have a genetic component, and **occurs only following second or subsequent contact with a particular antigen.** Hypersensitivity reactions were classified originally into a series of four types. In addition to those, a fifth type is also now included (Table 7.1) which meets all the criteria generally accepted of a hypersensitivity reaction. It is important to realize that *in vivo* the responses rarely happen in isolation. One antigen may stimulate responses of more than one type.

Table 7.1 *Characteristics of different types of hypersensitivity*

Type	Name	Response
I	Allergy	Antibody-mediated (IgE)
II	Cytotoxic	Antibody-mediated (non-IgE, to cell surfaces)
III	Immune complex	Antibody-mediated (non-IgE, to soluble molecules)
IV	Delayed	T cell mediated
V	Septicaemia	Cytokines

Type I hypersensitivity: allergy

This **immediate response** is also termed anaphylaxis or, commonly, allergy. Allergic diseases are among the major causes of illness and disability in the Western world. Allergic people are often sensitive to more than one substance. Antigens that cause allergic reactions are called **allergens** and they include:

- food;
- dust particles;
- medicines;
- insect venom;
- mould spores;
- pollen.

It is unclear why some individuals mount responses to certain antigens (allergens) and also why some people show a particularly strong response. It is possible that the tendency to be allergic is inherited, although not necessarily to any specific allergen. Children are much more likely to develop allergies if their parents have allergies. Even if only one parent is allergic, a child has a one in four chance of developing allergies. Exposure to allergens at certain times when the body's defences are lowered or weakened, such as after a viral infection, during puberty, or during pregnancy, seems to contribute to the development of allergies.

The basis of the Type I response is the production of IgE instead of other antibody isotypes. On initial contact with the allergen IgE is made, however the person shows no symptoms of an allergy. One particular cytokine (IL-4) is involved in the isotype switch from IgM to IgE. Although necessary, IL-4 is not in itself sufficient to cause a switch to IgE. A second signal, which can come from a variety of sources, is needed to complete the switch. Other cytokines are also thought to be active in the regulation of IgE production. IFN-γ, produced by Th1 helper cells, can antagonize the ability of IL-4 to induce IgE production. Recent studies have shown that T cells from **non-atopic** patients, (i.e. those not showing a skin reaction when exposed to allergen), when stimulated *in vitro* by specific allergen, produce primarily IFN-γ while T cells from atopic patients produce allergen-induced IL-4. Further, Th2 cells can produce IL-10 which can inhibit the production of cytokines such as IFN-γ. Thus IgE can be the prevalent antibody if Th2 rather than Th1 helper cells are stimulated in an atopic individual.

The initial response, i.e. on first exposure to a particular allergen, ends with IgE attached, via the Fc portion, to FcE receptors on tissue mast cells and circulating basophils (Figure 7.1). On the second encounter, and each subsequent encounter, with the same allergen this surface-bound IgE binds antigen in such a way that adjacent IgE molecules are cross-linked (Figure 7.2). Cross-linking of IgE causes the membrane-bound Fc receptors to move in the

Figure 7.1 *Following initial exposure to allergen, IgE binds to FcE receptors on tissue mast cells and circulating basophils*

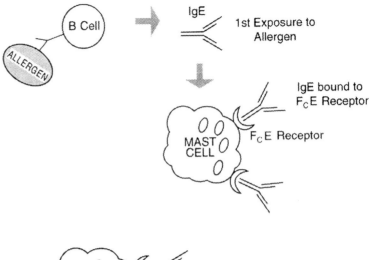

Figure 7.2 *On second, and subsequent, exposure to an allergen the binding surface-bound IgE to the allergen causes adjacent IgE molecules to be cross-linked. The FcE receptors can then move within the plane of the cell surface, causing degranulation leading to acute inflammation*

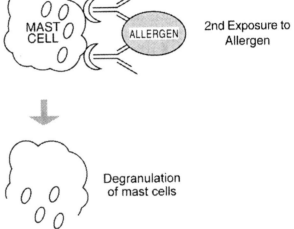

plane of the lipid membrane, a stimulus that causes the cell to degranulate and the granules to release their pre-formed inflammatory mediators. Histamine, one of the inflammatory mediators, binds to target receptors in the nose, lung, skin, gastrointestinal tract and near blood vessels via specific histamine receptors, especially H1 receptors. This activates a series of events leading to increased vascular permeability and dilation, stimulation of nerve fibres and initiation of inflammatory cascades that are collectively responsible for the signs and symptoms of immediate hypersensitivity, i.e. itching, sneezing, increased mucus secretion (rhinorrhoea), bronchospasm and, if enough vascular tissue is involved, hypotension.

Mast cells themselves both respond to and produce cytokines. Mast cells make IL-4 when stimulated. This may be particularly important in the propagation of IgE-producing B cells as well as the differentiation of T helper cells to the Th2 pathway, i.e. both conditions necessary for IgE production. In addition, IL-4 appears to be a secondary but important growth factor for mast cells. Eosinophils both respond to and manufacture certain cytokines. IL-5 appears to be a major growth factor for basophils and is also produced by Th2 cells. Thus an excess of allergen-specific Th2 activity could induce activation of each component of the allergic cascade and allergic disease might be considered to result from an imbalance between allergen-specific Th1 and Th2 activities.

Finally, activated basophils are known to secrete many cytokines such as IL-3, GM-CSF, TNF-α and IL-1. Any or all of these cytokines serve to enhance and sustain the allergic inflammatory process by mast cell activation (IL-3), further eosinophil recruitment (TNF-α), altering the target tissue (IL-1) and even direct tissue damage. The activated basophils also produce and secrete other protein and lipid mediators associated with allergic inflammation.

Overall, the events that comprise Type I hypersensitivity are analogous to those described previously for acute inflammation (Chapter 2) except that they tend to be more rapid and the symptoms induced are more severe. A strong determinant of the seriousness of the allergy, for the patient, is the site in the body where mast cell degranulation occurred. In the case of a reaction to an insect sting on the arm, for example, the response may be little more than a painful or itchy swelling. But, if the insect has been swallowed and the stinging occurs in the respiratory tract, the swelling could significantly affect breathing. A response to an inhaled allergen may provoke an allergic asthma attack. The symptoms of asthma include coughing, wheezing and shortness of breath due to a narrowing of the bronchial passages (airways) in the lungs and to excess mucus production. Asthma can be disabling and sometimes can be fatal. If wheezing and shortness of breath accompany allergy symptoms, it is a signal that the bronchial tubes also have become involved, indicating the need for medical attention.

Food allergies are believed to occur in 8% of children younger than 3 years old. Severe, life-threatening allergic reactions to food may occur as frequently as those to insect stings. A food allergy can cause symptoms involving a number of different body systems. For some people, food allergies can be life-threatening and others may have a mild reaction. Each individual's sensitivity will determine the degree to which the offending foods should be eliminated from the diet. The most common food allergens are:

- peanuts;
- fish;
- eggs;
- milk;
- wheat;
- soy.

During the last decade, the prevalence of asthma cases, hospitalizations, and deaths has been increasing. Members of ethnic minorities living in the inner cities in Western countries seem to be at particular risk for developing asthma. Asthma may be provoked both indoors and outdoors by house dust, animal proteins, fungal spores, pollens, moulds, house dust mite, etc. In gastrointestinal disease, the release of mediators causes a local inflammation which can either result in gastrointestinal symptoms or may allow absorption of antigenic material leading to systemic allergic reactions.

Milk, eggs and peanuts are three common food allergens. Cow's milk is one of the first foreign proteins encountered by infants. Cow's milk is a mixture of more than 20 protein components implicated in a number of possible immunologically mediated reactions. Chicken egg is a common food allergen particularly in children. The egg yolk has traditionally been considered less allergenic than the egg white. Ovalbumin, ovomucoid and ovotransferrin are the primary egg white allergens. Peanuts are one of the most allergenic foods ingested by children and adults. Unlike allergic reactions to milk and eggs, peanut allergies do not resolve with time.

The physicochemical properties that might account for the allergenicity of major food allergens are still to be investigated fully.

A number of allergic reactions have been grouped under the heading of 'restaurant syndromes'. These are reactions to monosodium glutamate (MSG), saurine and sulphites which can mimic anaphylaxis. Monosodium glutamate ingestion can produce flushing, chest pain, burning of the skin of the face, dizziness, sweating, palpitations, nausea, vomiting and headaches. Symptoms usually begin about 1 hour after the ingestion, but can be delayed up to 14 hours. About 15–20% of the population seem to be susceptible. Studies in patients experiencing episodes of anaphylaxis have failed to substantiate a relationship between MSG, or the ingestion of other food additives, and the production of such events. Spoiled fish contains saurine, a histamine-like chemical that, upon ingestion, produces symptoms identical to anaphylaxis. The ingestion of sulphites can, in some patients, produce a syndrome mimicking anaphylaxis.

Peanuts and shellfish are the most common foods that cause life-threatening allergies, although any food can be responsible for a severe or life-threatening allergic reaction.

The effects of airborne pollutants on the immune system have been widely studied in the respiratory tract. An airborne pollutant may enter the respiratory tract as a volatile gas (e.g. ozone, benzene), as liquid droplets (e.g. sulphuric acid, nitrogen dioxide), or as particulate matter (e.g. components of diesel exhaust, aromatic hydrocarbons). These pollutants may cause local and systemic hypersensitivities although, interestingly, the exposure may actually lead to immunosuppression. Most airborne pollutants are small molecular weight chemicals that must be coupled with other substances (e.g. proteins or conjugates) before they can be recognized by the immune system and cause an effect. Some hypersensitivity reactions (e.g. occupational asthma) can occur following exposure to toluene diisocyanate (frequently used in the petrochemical industry) and certain other volatile chemicals, while immunosuppression can be demonstrated following exposure to polycyclic aromatic hydrocarbons (e.g. 2,3,7,8-tetrachlordibenzo-p-dioxin). In addition to documenting systemic responses, more research is needed to learn about the effects of airborne pollutants on local mucosal immune responses in the gastrointestinal and respiratory tracts.

Anaphylactic shock is a dramatic allergic reaction that can result in collapse of the affected person and sometimes death. The onset is rapid and symptoms usually develop within 5–30 minutes of exposure to the allergen. Death may occur within a further 15 minutes. The precise frequency of occurrence of anaphylactic shock is unknown. However anecdotal evidence would indicate that it is increasing. Anaphylaxis can occur via any route of administration of antigen but episodes are more frequent and often more severe when antigen is injected rather than ingested. Often, the more rapid the onset, the more severe the episode. After oral administration there is often a delay, but symptoms usually occur within the first 2 hours. Nonetheless, in some cases, symptoms after oral ingestion can be almost immediate in onset and can be fatal.

Urticaria (itching), angioedema and flushing are the most common signs and symptoms of anaphylaxis. Frequently, the absence of such symptoms mitigate against the diagnosis of anaphylaxis although cardiovascular collapse with shock can occur immediately and without any cutaneous or respiratory symptoms in rare instances.

The next most common symptoms of anaphylactic shock are related to the respiratory tract. Early symptoms include: hoarseness or difficulty in breathing, weakness, paleness or swelling and redness of skin (often accompanied by hives), feeling of great anxiety, tingling feeling, dizziness and collapse. In addition, a diversity of other symptoms may also occur including: nausea, vomiting, intestinal cramps, diarrhoea, bloating, skin rash, hives, intense flushing, itching, swelling (especially at the site of an insect sting), swelling of throat and upper airway (blueness around nose and mouth), sudden runny nose, bronchospasm, wheezing, uncontrollable coughing, swelling of tongue, rapid heartbeat and low blood pressure. Two events participate in the production of shock symptoms. The first of these is **vasodilation** and the second is increased vascular permeability. Usually, the most significant of these is the increase in **vascular permeability**. This increase produces a shift of fluid from the intravascular to extravascular space and can result in rapid and profound losses of intravascular volume. Up to 50% of intravascular volume can be lost within 10 minutes. The biggest threat to life is constricted airways, which can cause death in minutes. The best possible treatment for allergy is avoidance of the known allergen. Unfortunately, this is not always possible. All persons with a known life-threatening allergy or a history of very severe symptoms are advised to own and carry with them an allergy kit or auto-injectable **adrenaline** kit. When the early symptoms are experienced the patient takes the pre-measured dose of adrenaline which pushes the blood pressure back to normal and reduces swelling (especially of the airways). It is the quickest and most effective way to stop the reaction.

The late phase in the Type I hypersensitivity response refers to the reappearance of symptoms after an apparent but temporary resolution. It is believed that these recurrent episodes are due to recruitment of other cells activated by chemotactic mediators released from mast cells and basophils. Unfortunately, however, during such episodes, there can be continuous release of histamine indicating that degranulation of mast cells and basophils may also be ongoing. In the case of a patient undergoing anaphylactic shock who has survived the initial onset of symptoms, death can occur at any time during the late phase.

> Flush reactions often mimic anaphylaxis, e.g. postmenopausal flush, alcohol-induced flush, idiopathic flush, flush due to medullary carcinoma of the thyroid, flush related to autonomic epilepsy and carcinoid syndrome.

Diagnosing allergies

When clinical examination would indicate that particular symptoms are the result of an allergy, a number of confirmatory tests can be carried out.

To confirm which allergen is responsible, skin testing may be recommended using extracts from allergens such as dust, pollens or moulds commonly found in the local area. A diluted extract of each kind of allergen is injected under the patient's skin or is applied to a scratch or puncture made on the patient's arm or back. A positive reaction (a small, raised, reddened area with a surrounding flush, called a wheal) is an important diagnostic clue but a positive reaction does not prove that a particular pollen is the cause of a patient's symptoms. Although such a reaction indicates that IgE antibody to a specific allergen is present in the skin, respiratory symptoms do not necessarily result. The demonstration of positive skin tests to specific allergens is known as **atopy**. The majority of those with allergy are also atopic.

Skin testing is not advisable in some people such as those with widespread skin conditions like eczema or if a patient has taken medications that interfere with skin testing. Diagnostic tests can be done using a blood sample from the patient to detect levels of IgE antibody to a particular allergen. One such blood test is called the **RAST (radioallergosorbent test)**. Unfortunately the RAST is expensive to perform, takes several weeks to yield results, and is somewhat less sensitive than skin testing. Overall, skin testing is the most sensitive and least costly diagnostic tool.

Treating allergic diseases

The three general approaches to the treatment of allergies are:

- avoidance of the allergen;
- medication to relieve symptoms;
- allergy immunization.

Although no cure for allergies has yet been found, one of these strategies or a combination of them can provide varying degrees of relief from allergy symptoms.

Complete **avoidance** of allergenic substances, although an extreme solution, may offer only temporary relief since a person who is sensitive to a chemical may subsequently develop allergies to new allergens after repeated exposure. For example, people allergic to ragweed may leave their ragweed-ridden communities and move to areas where ragweed does not grow, only to develop allergies to other weeds or even to grasses or trees in their new surroundings.

For people who find they cannot adequately avoid the allergens, the symptoms often can be controlled pharmacologically. Effective medications that can be prescribed include **antihistamines, topical nasal steroids and sodium cromoglycate**. Any of these can be used alone or in combination.

As the name indicates, an antihistamine counters the effects of histamine. Topical nasal steroids are anti-inflammatory drugs that stop the allergic reaction. In addition to other beneficial actions they reduce the number of mast cells in the nose and reduce mucus secretion and nasal swelling. The direct link between mast cell degranulation and allergy symptoms is apparent when mast cell membrane stabilizers are used as treatment. One such drug is sodium cromoglycate which inhibits the release of the mediators of anaphylaxis initiated by the interaction of antigen with IgE antibodies. Sodium cromoglycate interferes with the release of the inflammatory mediators but does not directly antagonize the mediators themselves. The drug is most effective when given prior to antigen challenge. Sodium cromoglycate has no antihistamine or anti-inflammatory activity. It is not a bronchodilator and has few general pharmacological effects. Patients with food allergies are advised to avoid the foods that provoke their symptoms, however patients unable to avoid allergenic foods under certain circumstances may be able to protect themselves against the effect of these foods by taking sodium cromoglycate shortly before a meal.

Immunotherapy, also called **desensitization** or **allergy immunization**, is the only available treatment that may reduce the patient's allergy symptoms in the long term. Patients receive injections of increasing concentrations of the allergen(s) to which they are sensitive. These injections reduce the amount of IgE antibodies and cause the production of IgG. About 85% of patients with allergic rhinitis (hay fever) will have a significant reduction in their hay fever symptoms and in their need for medication within 24 months of starting immunotherapy. Many patients are able to stop the injections with good, long-term results.

The recognition that allergy is associated with imbalanced Th1/Th2 activity may lead to cytokine-based therapies. Treatment agents could include cytokines themselves or pharmacological agents that can modulate specific cytokine profiles. Recombinant cytokines are being studied currently in a variety of allergic diseases. The limited use of these recombinant cytokines is due to at least three reasons: (a) they are extremely expensive, (b) they are extremely toxic, causing systemic side-effects such as fever, chills, muscle aches and fatigue and, in higher doses, they are potentially life threatening, and (c) giving large pharmacological doses of recombinant cytokines may create other imbalances in the host that could create other disease entities.

> The understanding of the allergen-specific Th1/Th2 imbalance and its importance in the pathophysiology of allergic diseases may facilitate improved clinical monitoring. Clinically useful laboratory assays could establish the Th2 nature of a specific response and then monitor response to therapy by watching for the change to a normal balance. Such concepts are currently being investigated as research related to allergic inflammation and cytokines continues to move steadily from bench to bedside.

Chemical sensitivity

'Allergic to the twentieth century' is a phrase that has been used to describe people who seem to react to everything in their environment. These allergy-like reactions can result from exposure to synthetic substances such as those found in paints or carpeting, or to natural substances, such as odours from plants and flowers. Although the symptoms may resemble those of true allergies, sensitivity to chemicals does not represent a true allergic reaction.

Type II hypersensitivity: antibody-dependent cell-mediated cytotoxicity

The antibody involved in this type of hypersensitivity is IgG or IgM, but not IgE. Antibody is produced in response to a cell surface and the cell is then lysed by complement and cleared by phagocytes. Clearly this is a beneficial response in the appropriate situation, for example when destroying infectious microorganisms. However it is not beneficial when targets are cells such as those entering the body in blood transfusions or tissue transplants. A model of Type II

Figure 7.3 *Rhesus incompatibility occurs when a woman who is Rhesus negative (Rh−) becomes pregnant with the child of a Rhesus positive (Rh+) father. The child will also be Rh+. If the Rh+ blood comes into contact with the mother's immune system she will produce antibodies against the baby's RBCs*

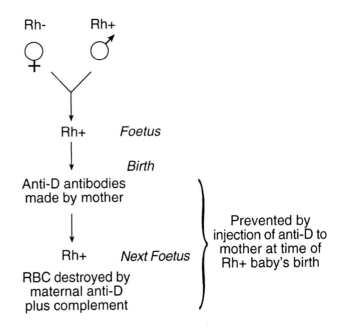

hypersensitivity is provided by the phenomenon of **Rhesus incompatibility**. This reaction is one which, formerly, caused considerable morbidity and mortality in newborn babies. Now, screening for this incompatibility is simple and routine and precautionary immunotherapy measures are highly effective.

Rhesus incompatibility occurs when a woman who is Rhesus negative (Rh−) becomes pregnant with the child of a Rhesus positive (Rh+) father (Figure 7.3). The Rh determinant is the **D antigen** present on erythrocytes. It is inherited as a dominant gene thus offspring of a Rh+ father will, themselves, often carry the D antigen. A Rh− woman's first pregnancy with a Rh+ baby should proceed normally. At the time of birth it is common that some of the baby's red blood cells (RBCs) will enter the maternal circulation. The mother is stimulated to mount an acquired response, leading to the synthesis of **anti-D antibodies**. During any subsequent pregnancy with a Rh+ child some of the anti-D antibodies will cross the placenta to the baby. A type II response then occurs which destroys the baby's erythrocytes. This condition is known as erythroblastosis foetalis, or **haemolytic disease of the newborn**. The affected baby may be stillborn, or if it is a live birth, immediate blood transfusion is the only effective treatment. In order to avoid this situation, pregnant women are screened for their blood type, including Rhesus status. At the time of delivery, Rh− women are given an injection of pre-formed anti-D antibody. This, with mother's complement, destroys the baby's Rh+ RBCs when they enter the circulation, before the mother's immune system can respond. Some of the administered anti-D may coat the RBCs, hiding the antigen from the immune system. Anti-D therapy must be repeated each time an affected mother gives birth. The antibodies pose no threat to subsequent babies as the amount given is small enough to ensure its rapid elimination from the circulation.

A transfusion of blood which is incompatible with the recipient's blood group, as defined by the ABO system, is destroyed by pre-existing antibodies in a Type II response. A new response may also be initiated against Class I or Class II MHC antigens on the surfaces of leukocytes in the case of a whole blood transfusion. The consequences for the individual of these responses can vary in severity according to several factors including:

- The amount of blood transfused.
- Whether the transfusion was of RBCs, of plasma only or of whole blood.
- Whether the patient had previously received similarly mis-matched whole blood. (In the latter case, antibodies to MHC antigens may already be in existence within the recipient so causing a rapid, secondary response.)

In the case of incompatible tissue transplants, antibodies are directed against MHC Class I antigens on tissue cells and MHC Class I and Class II on any leukocytes that may be included in the transplanted tissue. Circulating leukocytes are generally removed from transplant tissues, e.g. by perfusion with saline, as they may increase significantly the risk of rejection. The reason for this is that foreign MHC Class II antigens are very potent stimulators of T cells. Once again a previous mis-matched transplant or whole blood transfusion may have induced antibodies thereby increasing the speed and effectiveness of the response. This is known as hyperacute rejection and signs of it may be present within minutes of the re-establishment of blood circulation to the transplant.

Type III hypersensitivity: immune complex disease

This hypersensitivity also involves antibodies, predominantly IgG and IgM, but not IgE. Responses are directed against **soluble antigens** and the pathological sequelae usually result from **immune complex formation** and deposition (Figure 7.4). The antibodies are usually of low affinity. Pathologies may also be associated with complement deficiencies. This linkage is thought to operate by the decreased removal of immune complexes because of the absence of sufficient complement molecules to interact with phagocyte complement receptors.

An early example of Type III hypersensitivity was observed with passive immunization for diphtheria. Patients were given doses of pre-formed horse antibodies. When injected, these antibodies

Figure 7.4 *Type III hypersensitivity responses produce antibodies directed against soluble antigens, forming immune complexes. These are deposited on endothelial surfaces in many parts of the body*

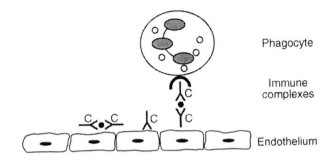

Figure 7.5 *Immune complexes deposited on endothelial surfaces attract phagocytes. Failing to complete phagocytosis of the host cells, the phagocyte releases lysosomal enzymes and reactive oxygen species directly onto the tissue, causing damage. Further inflammatory responses are also stimulated*

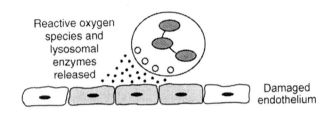

A Type III hypersensitivity response similar to farmer's lung, and affecting workers indoors, is humidifier fever. In the 1950s, studies established a relationship between malaise, cough, shortness of breath and contaminated humidifiers, whether these are personal humidifiers or in air-conditioning systems. Illness commonly occurs when a worker returns to work after a period away from work and symptoms are those of an influenza-like illness, sometimes called 'Monday sickness'! Humidifier fever is thought to be a response to viable cells, spores, dead cellular material (proteins, polysaccharides). Spores and dead cellular material are typically less than 0.5 μ in diameter and therefore capable of penetrating deep into the lungs.

tackled the diphtheria organisms: however they themselves were foreign to the affected patients. Antibody-mediated immune responses were stimulated. The new antibodies bound with low affinity to the horse antibodies forming small immune complexes. These were deposited from the circulation primarily in the skin, joints, lungs and glomerulus of the kidney. The deposited complexes attracted phagocytes which attempted to phagocytose the tissue cells that had been 'opsonized'. Failing to complete phagocytosis, these cells released lysosomal enzymes and reactive oxygen species directly onto the tissue (Figure 7.5). Thus many tissues sustained damage and their function was impaired. This condition was known as **serum sickness**. Passive immunization is now employed only in a very limited range of situations, for example, where the patient is pregnant or immunosuppressed so cannot withstand exposure to an active immunogen, and great care is taken to avoid the induction of serum sickness.

The conditions which predispose to Type III hypersensitivity are those where low affinity antibody is produced in low amounts over a period of time. Antigens which satisfy these criteria include some environmental antigens to which people may be exposed constantly over prolonged periods, e.g. in occupational environments. One of these is the mould *Saccharomycetes* which is found in hay and induces the condition known as **farmer's lung or hypersensitivity pneumonitis**.

A second stimulant of low affinity antibody is thought to be self antigens, leading to autoimmune diseases (Chapter 8). Self antigens are components of the host which, for reasons that are not yet clearly understood, induce an immune response. Because they are part of the host, the antigens cannot be eliminated so immune complex production does not stop.

Type IV hypersensitivity: delayed type (DTH)

This type of response does not involve antibody. Its defining characteristic is that it should be transferred from one animal to an unaffected animal by transfer of T cells. Thus T cells are the central regulatory component. When involved in Type IV responses the T cell is known as T_{DTH} (T cell of delayed-type hypersensitivity). Within the Type IV response there are four different phenomena which rarely occur separately. These are:

- Jones–Mote reaction;
- contact hypersensitivity;
- tuberculin reaction;
- granulomatous reaction.

Contact hypersensitivity

The characteristic feature of this response is the induction of localized **eczema** following contact with an allergen. The most common allergens to provoke contact hypersensitivity are nickel, chromate, rubber products and chemicals contained in poison ivy. What these substances all have in common is that they contain microscopic particles, termed **haptens**, that can enter the epidermis of intact skin. There they are conjugated to normal body proteins. This conjugation has the effect of making the haptens more antigenic because several haptens can bind to a single protein, thus increasing both the dose and the size of the antigen. The protein–hapten complex is presented to T cells by epidermal antigen-presenting cells (APCs), predominantly **Langerhans cells**. Local **keratinocytes** may also act as APCs and as sources of a wide range of pro-inflammatory cytokines and chemokines. These molecules attract further leukocytes to the site and promote Langerhans cell activity. The subsequent T-cell response is not confined to the local epidermis because the Langerhans cells can enter the many lymphatics that drain the skin and travel to adjacent lymph nodes. In the lymph nodes they are known as **dendritic cells or interdigitating cells**.

The initial activation of T cells that occurs in the paracortical areas of the lymph nodes does not produce any symptoms, however, by analogy with Type I hypersensitivity, the affected individual is said to be sensitized. On subsequent contact with the allergen these T cells will be stimulated to mount a swifter, more effective secondary response. Meanwhile, back at the site of initial contact with the allergen, mast cells have degranulated and released inflammatory mediators and pro-inflammatory cytokines. An inflammatory response then ensues, however the principal leukocyte type infiltrating the skin is not the neutrophil but mononuclear leukocytes. Infiltration is likely to be underway within 4 hours of contact with allergen and macrophage numbers peak at about 72 hours. Thereafter the response clears, promoted by down-regulatory cytokines such as transforming growth factor β (TGF-β), IL-10 and prostaglandin E (PGE) released by the macrophages, lymphocytes and adjacent keratinocytes.

The response that is known as the **Jones–Mote reaction** is also induced by contact with allergen but is characterized by the infiltration of basophils into the inflammatory site. The factors which cause this particular component of the reaction are unknown.

Tuberculin reaction

This type of hypersensitivity is the basis of the widely used Tuberculin Skin Test (TST), also called the Mantoux Test. This test involves the inoculation of an individual with **purified protein derivative (PPD)** and is the standard method for detecting infection by *Mycobacterium tuberculosis*. The reaction is measured as millimetres of **induration (hard swelling)** of the skin after 48–72 hours.

The basis of the tuberculin response is the re-activation of antigen-specific memory T cells within the dermal layer of the skin. The T cells produce TNF-β (lymphotoxin) which act on local vascular endothelial cells to induce the infiltration of neutrophils into the skin. By about 12 hours the predominant infiltrating cell types are mononuclear leukocytes: lymphocytes and monocytes, and their number reaches a peak at about 48 hours. By this time the infiltrate also involves the epidermis. The characteristic indurations are a result of the combination of a large number of cells with oedema. The signs of the reaction normally last for between 5 and 7 days after which they resolve. This is in contrast to the situation where, if there is a constant source of antigen as a result of infection, the reaction progresses to become a granulomatous lesion.

Since TST is the only way to determine asymptomatic infection by *M. tuberculosis*, the false-negative rate cannot be calculated. A negative TST does not rule out TB disease in a child. Approximately 10% of otherwise normal children with culture-proven TB do not react to tuberculin initially. Most of these children have reactive skin tests during treatment, which suggests that TB contributes to the immunosuppression that prevented the skin reaction. In most cases, the anergy (non-reactivity) occurs to all antigens but, in some cases, reactions to tuberculin are negative while reactions to other antigens remain positive. The rate of false-negative TST is higher in those who are:

- tested soon after becoming infected with TB;
- in children with debilitating or immunosuppressive illnesses, malnutrition, or viral and certain bacterial infections;
- in infants.

Poor technique can also influence the false-positive rate. The rate of false-negative TST in children with TB who are infected with human immunodeficiency virus (HIV) is unknown, but it is certainly higher than 10%. The clinician cannot know immediately which exposed children are infected because the development of DTH to tuberculin may take up to 3 months. Unfortunately, in children under 5 years of age, severe TB, especially meningeal and disseminated disease, can occur in under 3 months, before the TST becomes reactive.

False-positive reactions to TST are often attributed to asymptomatic infection by environmental non tuberculous mycobacteria. Vaccination with *M. bovis* can cause transient reactivity to a subsequent TST, but the association is weak. Most, up to 90%, children who received BCG as infants have a non-reactive TST at 5 years of age. **BCG, or Bacillus–Calmette–Guerin**, is the vaccine for TB still given to children in many Western countries. Among older children or adolescents who receive BCG, most develop a reactive skin test initially; however, by 10–15 years post-vaccination, 80–90% have lost tuberculin reactivity. Many recipients of BCG have a reactive TST because they are infected with *M. tuberculosis* and are at risk for disease, especially if they have had recent contact with an infectious TB patient. In general, TST reaction should be interpreted in the same manner for persons who have received BCG and for unvaccinated persons.

Granulomatous reaction

This type of DTH has the most severe consequences for the individual because of the presence of often extensive tissue damage. An alternative name for **granulomatous** hypersensitivity is **chronic inflammation**. A clear distinction can be drawn between persistent acute inflammation and chronic inflammation on the basis of the cell types persisting at the site of the lesion. With acute inflammation, no matter how long-lasting it may be, the predominant infiltrating cells are neutrophils. By contrast the hallmark of chronic inflammation is mononuclear cells: monocytes, macrophages and lymphocytes. The conditions that predispose to development of the potentially more damaging chronic disease, rather than to recurrent acute episodes, are unknown. One probable contributing factor is diminished T-cell function.

There are two types of granuloma:

- **foreign-body granulomas** are initiated by inert foreign bodies; whereas

Figure 7.6 *An immune granuloma is a benign tissue growth that begins with macrophages. Many of the macrophages contain ingested foreign organisms that they have not been able to kill. The macrophages develop into multi-nucleated giant cells. Lymphocytes and epitheloid cells are also present. Fibroblasts are attracted and secrete the connective tissue that forms the tough outer layer*

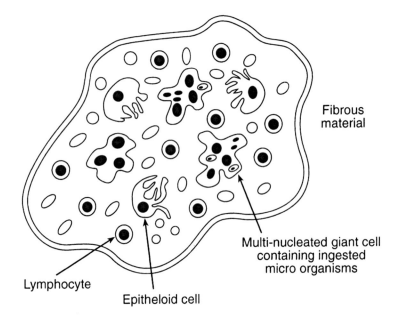

Fibrous material

Multi-nucleated giant cell containing ingested micro organisms

Lymphocyte

Epitheloid cell

- **immune granulomas** represent a T cell-mediated reaction to immunogenic particles.

An immune granuloma (Figure 7.6) is a benign tissue growth that begins with macrophages, which have often ingested foreign antigen that they have not been able to kill. Lymphocytes are also present. The macrophages then develop into **multi-nucleated giant cells.** Another cell type is **epitheloid cells,** of uncertain origin. The processes that occur are analogous to wound healing, except of course that there is no wound to heal. Macrophage cytokines are secreted that attract fibroblasts to the site. Fibroblast adhesion and proliferation are also promoted, e.g. by fibroblast growth factor (FGF). The final stage in granuloma formation is the production of collagen by the fibroblasts which forms a mesh of strong connective tissue around the granuloma. Once complete, the granuloma is impenetrable to other cells or molecules so the immune response is unable to clear it. Eventually the cells in the central area of the granuloma become necrotic. Despite this, viable organisms may remain and it is their re-activation, causing rupture of the granuloma and spread to other tissues, that can be devastating for the patient. The impairment of tissue function is caused by the presence of many tough granulomata which occupy the space of normal tissue and inhibit its function. Two examples of diseases involving granulomatous reactions are **leprosy and tuberculosis (TB).** Both of these are of infectious origin; the causative organisms are *M. leprae* and *M. tuberculosis*, respectively.

Leprosy (**Hansen's disease**) exists in two forms depending on the status of the infected person's immune response. If the response mediated by T cells and macrophages is compromised, granulomata form in the skin. This is called lepromatous leprosy. On the other hand, when these cell-mediated responses are intact, Schwann cells of the nerves are the primary target of the organism (tuberculoid leprosy). In fact, these are two poles of a spectrum of disease manifestations. Between the two poles are patients with intermediate features as seen in the borderline lepromatous and borderline tuberculoid forms. Humoral immunity is present throughout the spectrum but does not seem to provide protection. The accumulation of leukocytes causes intra-neural pressure to increase, effectively blocking the tiny blood vessels supplying the nerves. This causes the destruction of the nerves which is a feature of tuberculoid leprosy. Where the sensory nerves are destroyed, this can result in loss of feeling, particularly in the extremities, i.e. hands and feet. These areas are then prone to ulceration damage due, for example, to handling hot utensils and walking on unprotected feet. Where the motor nerves are affected, various forms of paralysis develop, such as 'dropped foot', 'dropped wrist', 'clawed hand' and 'lagophthalmos' (eyes can't close, due to seventh cranial nerve involvement). Many leprosy patients become blind due to paralysis of the fifth cranial nerve which may produce corneal anaesthesia. The insensitive cornea is then vulnerable to injury and sight may be lost. Damage to the autonomic nervous system can result in the sweat and sebaceous glands becoming inoperative causing dryness and cracking of the skin which can lead to secondary infection and consequent ulceration.

Over the past decade, the incidence of TB in both developed and developing countries has increased dramatically. According to World Health Organization (WHO) estimates, in 1990 there were 8 million new cases of TB and 3 million deaths due to the disease worldwide; 1.3 million new cases and 450 000 deaths were among children under 15 years of age. WHO projects that 90 million new cases and 30 million deaths, including 4.5 million deaths among children, will occur in the 1990s. One of the major reasons for the rise in incidence of TB is the increase in the number of people with compromised immune systems due to HIV infections. For individuals with normal immune systems who are tuberculin positive, the risk of developing TB sometime during their lives is 10%. For people who are HIV positive, that risk is 50%.

For over 40 years the standard drug for treating TB has been **isoniazid (INH)**. Studies have shown that it is 60–90% effective in preventing TB when it is taken over 6–12 months. However, INH has significant drawbacks. It must be taken for a substantial length of time and, unfortunately, some strains of M. *tuberculosis* have become INH resistant, especially in HIV positive people. An alternative therapy, that could be given for a shorter period of time, is now needed so that patients would be more likely to comply.

In the male leprosy patient, destruction of the testes may lead to hormonal imbalance. The sufferer may acquire female characteristics and this stigma is enhanced when the victim also suffers from destruction of the larynx, resulting in a squeaky, husky, female type voice. Paradoxically, the disease is not usually fatal and M. *leprae* is one of the least infectious organisms. Thus the biblical fear of lepers is based more on the physical appearance and possible feminization of patients.

Although cases among children represent a small percentage of all TB cases, infected children are a reservoir from which many adult cases will arise. TB diagnosis in children usually follows discovery of a case in an adult, and relies on tuberculin skin testing, chest radiograph, and clinical signs and symptoms. However, clinical symptoms are nonspecific, skin testing and chest radiographs can be difficult to interpret, and routine laboratory tests are not helpful. Although more rapid and sensitive laboratory testing, which takes into account recent advances in biomedical science, is being developed, the results have been disappointing. Better techniques would especially benefit children and infants in whom early diagnosis is imperative for preventing progressive TB.

In developing countries, the risk for TB infection and disease is relatively uniform in the population. In industrialized countries, risk is more uneven and depends on the individual's past or present activities and their exposure to persons at high risk for the disease (Table 7.2).

The natural history of TB in children follows a continuum; however, it is useful to consider three basic stages: exposure, infection and disease. If a child is infected, it is usually because he/she was in close contact with an infected person. In adults, the distinction between TB infection and disease is usually clear because most disease is caused by reactivation of dormant organisms years after infection.

Crohn's Disease is a chronic granulomatous disease of the terminal ileum of the large intestine. The known mycobacterial involvement with other granulomatous diseases leads researchers to continue to look for other mycobacteria as potential causes. Crohn's disease is characterized by ulceration and fistula formation. Unlike in TB, the granulomas usually do not have caseation

---

Table 7.2

People at high risk for *Mycobacterium tuberculosis* infection in industrialized countries include:

- Close contacts of a person with infectious tuberculosis (TB);
- People from high-incidence areas (e.g. Asia, Africa, Latin America);
- The elderly;
- Residents of long-term care facilities;
- Intravenous drug users;
- People who may have occupational exposure to TB.

People at high risk of developing TB once infected include:

- HIV-positive people;
- Other immunosuppressed people, e.g. through immunosuppressive treatments post-transplantation, viral infections or malnutrition;
- People with a history of inadequately treated TB;
- Infants.

necrosis. Acid-fast stains and cultures are negative. For these reasons, *M. tuberculosis* has not been considered in the aetiology of Crohn's disease. Nonetheless, epidemiological data would strongly suggest an infectious aetiology for Crohn's disease. Polymerase chain reaction (PCR) and immunological techniques have greatly enhanced the ability of researchers to detect micro-organisms in patient specimens, although different laboratories often yield conflicting results. Within the gut there are many non-pathogenic commensal organisms so distinguishing those which do have a causative role in gut pathologies is a significant challenge.

Type V hypersensitivity: septic shock

Septic shock, also known as **septicaemia** or **endotoxaemia**, is most commonly caused by endotoxins found as components of Gram-negative bacterial cell walls. Septic shock may also be induced by Gram-positive bacteria. The most powerful stimulant of this syndrome is **lipopolysaccharide**, a component of certain bacterial cell walls (**LPS**, Figure 7.7). The LPS molecule is complex but the precise immunostimulant is thought to be the lipid core, the **lipid A**. Following interaction with cell surface molecules, including CD14, a wide range of immunological responses is triggered. The LPS is a potent stimulus of the pro-inflammatory cytokines TNF-α, IL-1 and

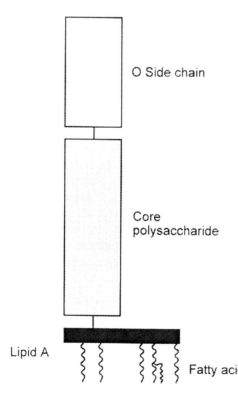

Figure 7.7 *Lipopolysacchride (LPS) from the cell walls of Gram-negative bacteria*

IL-6 which are released by macrophages. IL-1, with TNF-α and IFN-γ, causes tachycardia and hypotension. Tumour necrosis factor increases the procoagulant activity of endothelial cells and the expression of adhesion molecules. These events facilitate the accumulation of inflammatory cells.

Management of the shock-specific symptoms is still one of the most challenging problems faced by microbiologists and clinicians. The symptoms include hypotension, insufficient tissue perfusion, uncontrollable bleeding and multisystem organ failure caused mainly by hypoxia, tissue acidosis and severe local alterations of metabolism. The development of septicaemia is frequently recognized only at a relatively late stage when there is a drop in blood pressure. The massive deterioration of haemostasis, also known as **disseminated intravascular coagulation (DIC)**, involves blood vessels, platelets, blood coagulation and fibrinolytic processes, the presence or absence of inhibitors, the kallikrein–kininogen system, and complement.

One possible indicator of a lethal outcome of bacterial sepsis is a serum TNF-α concentration above 1 ng/mL. However absolute serum concentrations of pro-inflammatory cytokines are normally not reliable indicators of the severity of the patient's condition and are not predictive of the clinical outcome.

One example of septic shock is the so-called **toxic shock syndrome (TSS)** which is observed mainly in younger women. It is caused by tampons contaminated with *Staphylococcus aureus*. These bacteria produce an exotoxin of 23.1 kDa, TSST-1 (toxic shock syndrome toxin), which induces the synthesis of IL-1 and TNF-α. Specific neutralizing antibodies directed against bacterial endotoxins inactivate the bacterial toxin. However such antibodies are of prophylactic value only and cannot be used to treat acute cases. Animal experiments with genetically engineered **IL-1 receptor antagonist (IL-1RA)** have shown that this IL-1 inhibitor positively influences blood pressure, initial leukopaenia and later leukocytosis in septic shock. There is hope that, in humans, the administration of cytokine inhibitors may reduce the high mortality rates associated with septic shock. Unfortunately clinical trials with cytokine inhibitors have not lived up to expectations. Part of the reason for this may be that, in inhibiting the pathological effects of cytokines, the patient is also deprived of their beneficial effects. Genetically engineered cytokine inhibitors may, some day, be able specifically to regulate cytokine levels and functions so that only the pathogenic effects are inhibited.

Suggested further reading

Giegler, A., Sinha, B., Hartmann, G. and Endres, S. (1997) Taming TNF: strategies to restrain this proinflammatory cytokine. *Immunology Today* **18**, 487–492.

Grewe, M., Bruijnzeel-Koomen, C.A.F.M., Schopf, E., Thepen, T., Langeveld-Wildschut, A.G., Ruzicka, T. and Krutman, J. (1998) A role for Th1 and Th2 cells in the immunopathogenesis of atopic dermatitis. *Immunology Today* **19**, 359–361.

Gutierez-Ramos, J.C. and Bluethmann H. (1997) Molecules and mechanisms operating in septic shock: lessons from knockout mice. *Immunology Today* **18**, 329–334.

Hamilton, G. (1998) Let them eat dirt. *New Scientist* **159**, 26–31.

Pretolani, M. and Goldman, M. (1997) IL-10: a potential therapy for allergic inflammation? *Immunology Today* **18**, 277–280.

Ridley, M. (1999) *Genome*. London: Fourth Estate.

Self-assessment questions

1. Explain why Fc receptors can be specific for IgE.
2. What is atopy?
3. Explain the current understanding of the link between CD4$^+$ T cell types and IgE.
4. Why is adrenaline an effective treatment for anaphylactic shock?
5. Why is a Rh− woman given a small amount of anti-D antibody when giving birth to Rh+ babies?
6. When does hyperacute rejection occur?
7. List three conditions that may be associated with Type III hypersensitivity.
8. Within the immune system, what are dendritic cells?
9. Distinguish between the two forms of Hansen's Disease (leprosy).
10. What component of Gram +ve bacteria is considered responsible for the induction of cytokine release during Type V hypersensitivity?

Key Concepts and Facts

Hypersensitivity
- Involves inappropriate immune responses.
- Is classified into five types.

Type I Hypersensitivity
- Is commonly known as allergy.
- Is an immediate response involving IgE.
- Initial encounter with antigen (allergen) causes sensitization, i.e. IgE bound to FcE receptors on mast cells.
- Symptoms occur on second and subsequent encounters with an allergen.
- In some individuals very rapid and severe responses cause anaphylactic shock that may be fatal.

Type II Hypersensitivity
- Is known as cytotoxic hypersensitivity.
- Involves immediate antibody-mediated (IgG or IgM) responses against cells.
- Causes destruction of cells in mismatched blood transfusions or transplanted tissues.
- Underlies Rhesus incompatibility.

Type III Hypersensitivity
- Is known as immune complex-mediated hypersensitivity.
- Involves immediate antibody-mediated (IgG or IgM) responses against soluble proteins.
- Occurs in response to persistent exposure to weakly immunogenic antigens.
- Antigens may be self components, leading to autoimmune diseases.

Type IV Hypersensitivity
- Involves delayed cell-mediated responses.
- Is characterized by a range of different responses.
- Granuloma formation is the most damaging type of response, leading to significant pathology, e.g. in tuberculosis or leprosy.

Type V Hypersensitivity
- Is also known as septicaemia or septic shock.
- Involves exaggerated natural responses, i.e. inflammation.
- Is characterized by the production of high concentrations of the pro-inflammatory cytokines IL-1, IL-6 and TNF-α.
- Is responsible for significant mortality in hospital intensive care units.

Chapter 8
Autoimmune disease

Learning objectives

After studying this chapter you should confidently be able to:

Describe the spectrum of responses that underlie autoimmune diseases.

Describe the principal signs and symptoms associated with a range of autoimmune diseases.

Discuss current concepts of the causes of autoimmune diseases.

Normal immune responses are not directed against host tissues. This is a result of the elimination of potentially self-reactive T cells in the thymus. However, contrary to this supposed central tenet of modern immunology is the observation that self-directed antibodies occur in the circulation of healthy individuals. This is most marked in older people, over age 65 years. While such antibodies are believed not to be associated with any disease process, their existence is not fully explicable given our current understanding of self-tolerance. In **autoimmune diseases**, on the other hand, antibodies or T cells directed against self, the so-called **autoantibodies or autoreactive T cells**, are thought to be causally associated with a range of different pathologies.

Autoimmune diseases affect some 5–7% of adults in Europe and North America. They have a major socio-economic impact as they are associated with debilitation during the most productive years of life yet do not shorten life expectancies. In the 1950s criteria were defined against which, it was thought, a diagnosis of autoimmune disease would be made in the future. These included:

- detection of autoantibody or autoreactive cells;
- identification of the corresponding antigen;
- induction of an analogous response in an experimental animal.

Experience of the past 40 years has shown that these proposals were rather overly-optimistic. Current criteria should take into account:

- the fact that autoimmune responses may be normal physiological events;
- the identification, to date, of only an extremely small number of involved antigens (autoantigens);
- the histocompatibility barriers that make it impossible to transfer the diseases directly from humans to experimental animals.

When autoantibodies or autoreactive cells are found in an individual with detectable pathology, there may be several possible explanations for the observations. Firstly, the autoantibodies or cells may have caused the lesions; secondly some other event may have caused the lesions which then led to an autoimmune response or, finally, one particular factor may have caused both the lesions and the autoimmune response.

A diagnosis of autoimmune disease based on clinical and laboratory findings is strengthened by any of the following criteria:

- Other autoimmune diseases have been diagnosed in the same individual or the same family.
- The patient expresses an MHC haplotype for which there is a statistical association with an autoimmune disease.
- A biopsy specimen of the target organs show infiltration with lymphocytes expressing a restricted range of V gene types (i.e. many of the lymphocyte receptors (TCR or Ig) recognize a single epitope. In a normal response to non-self TCR and Ig are directed against a spectrum of different epitopes).
- There is aberrant expression of MHC Class II antigens on the affected organ.
- There is a favourable response to treatment by immunosuppression, e.g. immunosuppressive drugs.

Autoimmune diseases are divided broadly into two types:

- organ specific diseases;
- non-organ specific, or systemic, diseases.

In practice, a continuum of diseases exists, many showing characteristics of both extreme forms of disease. Figure 8.1 shows the spectrum of autoimmune diseases. This classification is based not so much on the location of the disease symptoms, as the target site for the immune response. Thus in organ-specific diseases the response is targeted against a single organ or tissue while in non-organ specific the target antigen is found systemically throughout the body.

Non-organ specific autoimmune diseases

Rheumatoid arthritis (RA) is probably the best-known of the

It is an interesting fact that patients with one organ-specific autoimmune disease have an increased risk of getting a second disease of this type, while their risk of getting a non-organ specific disease is not increased. The risk-pattern for patients with a non-organ specific disease is similarly related to their disease type. This may indicate a different underlying mechanism for each type of disease.

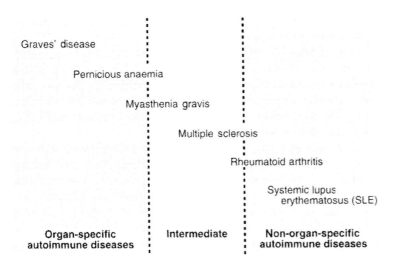

Figure 8.1 *The spectrum of autoimmune diseases ranges from organ-specific diseases to non-organ-specific diseases. Intermediate diseases display features of both types*

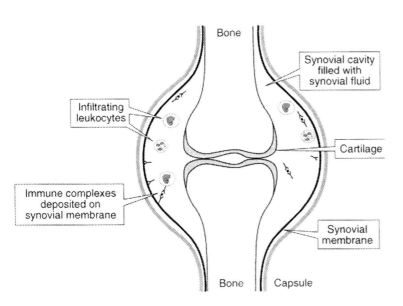

Figure 8.2 *Rheumatoid arthritis (RA) is a heterogeneous group of disorders characterized by immune-mediated inflammation of the synovium of the joints*

autoimmune diseases. Rheumatoid arthritis is, in fact, a heterogeneous group of disorders characterized by immune-mediated inflammation of the synovium of joints (Figure 8.2). Its incidence shows a distinct gender bias with about 5% of women and 2% of men in Britain affected; similar figures in the USA mean that about 4 million people have this condition. The incidence of RA also increases with age such that it affects some 25% of patients over 70.

The most common association with the onset of RA is the presence of IgM antibodies directed against antigenic determinants on the Fc portion of IgG. This autoantibody is known as **Rheumatoid Factor (RF)** and is present in 75% of patients with chronic RA. The dilemma is that RF is not present in all RA patients and its level in the serum does not always correlate with disease severity. A finding of RF alone is not diagnostic of RA because RF may be positive in a number of conditions besides RA including chronic liver disease, sarcoidosis, chronic pulmonary disease, other rheumatoid conditions and in infections such as syphilis and EBV/CMV. Further, infusion of RF-laden plasma into volunteers does not induce RA in them.

The predominant symptoms of RA are associated with the joints of the hands and feet, although other joints may also become involved. In RA the joints tend to be involved in a symmetrical pattern. That is, if knuckles on the right hand are inflamed, it is likely that knuckles on the left hand will be inflamed as well. Affected joints never appear red unless there is secondary disease, e.g. infection. Patients may have symptoms such as morning stiffness or stiffness following periods of inactivity, fatigue and weight loss. For some 10% of patients the onset is abrupt.

Analysis of affected joints shows that large amounts of **immune complexes** are present in the joint fluid. These complexes may include both RF–IgG and collagen–anticollagen. The joint synovium contains large numbers of neutrophils, normally absent from joints. Some of the neutrophils may contain phagocytosed IgM, IgG and complement. The inflammatory process within the joint is maintained by the neutrophils which release degradative enzymes including elastase; cathepsins (break down proteoglycan); glycosidases and collagenases. Also released are activators of the complement, kinin, clotting and fibrinolytic cascades. Myeloperoxidase sustains the production of reactive oxygen species (ROS) and these, together with prostaglandins, leukotrienes, platelet-activating factor (PAF) and complement factors C3a and C4a maintain the symptoms of the inflammation and attract further neutrophils. Monocytes are also present and release similar mediators to the neutrophils. Lymphocytes and plasma cells are seen to be present in germinal centres.

The synovial membrane responds to the ongoing events by proliferating and developing an enhanced vascular supply. The exact cause of this is uncertain. The term **pannus** is variously applied to proliferative synovium or to the fibrous scar that develops at the same location. Some patients may show a systemic vasculitis (inflammation of blood vessel walls), with IgM, IgG and complement in vessel walls. Usually there are large amounts of circulating immune complexes and apparent complement deficiency due to its constant activation and consumption.

There is a genetic component in the occurrence of RA. Its incidence amongst first degree relatives, i.e. parents, children and siblings, is reported to be twice that expected by chance and the prevalence of **seropositivity** (RF positivity) in unaffected family members may be higher. Concordance is 30% in dizygotic twins and 95% in monozygotic twins.

There are three major goals in the treatment of RA. These are:

- reduction of inflammation and pain;
- maintenance of joint function;
- prevention of deformity.

Anti-inflammatory and analgesic drugs can help reduce inflammation and pain while the second and third goals are more difficult to attain. The first-line drugs include **non-steroidal anti-inflammatory drugs (NSAIDs)** which are sufficient to manage 50–70% of RA patients. Second-line drugs include gold salts and the chelator D-penicillamine. In contrast to the NSAIDs, these drugs are disease-modifying, i.e. some patients go into remission, perhaps due to an immunosuppressive action. Unfortunately their use is limited by their toxicities. The use of immunosuppressive drugs such as cyclophosphamide or methotrexate is restricted to only about 5% of RA patients whose disease has not responded well to other drugs. These cause **generalized immunosuppression** with the attendant problems of susceptibility to infection. For people with hips or knees that have been severely damaged by the disease process, total joint replacement can allow them to lead an independent life.

Multiple sclerosis (MS) is a chronic disease of the central nervous system (CNS) and one of the most common causes of chronic neurological disability in young adults. The chronic–progressive form of the disease often leads to a complete loss of the ability to walk within 2 years of onset and total disability after 8–10 years. The disease is characterized by:

- weakness or paralysis in the limbs;
- vertigo and incontinence.

Symptoms of acute disease include:

- muscle wasting;
- progressive visual failure;
- epilepsy and aphasia.

The underlying pathological process in this autoimmune disease is the attack by specific T cells (autoreactive T cells) on nerve cells (Figure 8.3). Components of myelin such as **myelin basic protein (MBP)** have been the focus of much research because, when injected into laboratory animals, they can precipitate **experimental allergic encephalomyelitis (EAE)**, a chronic relapsing brain and spinal cord disease that resembles MS. The injected myelin probably stimulates the immune system to produce anti-myelin T cells that attack the animal's own myelin. Abnormalities or malfunctions in the blood–brain barrier, a protective membrane that controls the passage of substances from the blood into the CNS, may be present in MS allowing components of the immune system to get through the barrier and cause damage. Confusingly, the existence of autoreactive

> The laboratory diagnosis of RA involves:
>
> - a full blood count showing anaemia with mild leukocytosis, eosinophilia and thrombocytosis;
> - an elevated erythrocyte sedimentation rate (ESR);
> - serum containing RF of IgM, or, occasionally, IgG, isotype.

Figure 8.3 *The underlying pathological process in multiple sclerosis (MS) is the attack by specific T cells (autoreactive T cells) on nerve cells*

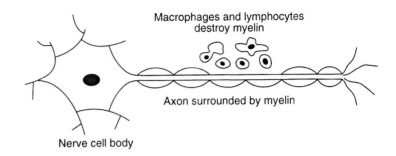

T cells or autoantibodies to myelin is not sufficient for MS to occur as both may be detected in healthy individuals.

There seems to be little doubt that something in the environment is involved in triggering MS. In addition, increasing scientific evidence suggests that genetics may play a role in determining a person's susceptibility to MS. Some ethnic populations, such as Gypsies, Eskimos and Bantus, never get MS. Native Indians of North and South America, the Japanese, and other Asian peoples have very low incidence rates. It is unclear whether this is due mostly to genetic or environmental factors.

In the population at large, the chance of developing MS is less than 0.1%. However, if one person in a family has MS, that person's first-degree relatives have a 1–3% chance of getting the disease. For identical twins, the likelihood that the second twin may develop MS if the first twin does is about 30%; for dizygotic twins, the likelihood is similar to that for non-twin siblings, at about 4%. The fact that the rate for identical twins both developing MS is significantly less than 100% suggests that the disease is not entirely genetically controlled. Some, but definitely not all, of this effect may be due to shared exposure to something in the environment, or to the fact that some people with MS lesions remain essentially asymptomatic throughout their lives.

There is as yet no cure for MS. Many patients do well with no therapy at all. Naturally occurring or spontaneous remissions make it difficult to determine therapeutic effects of experimental treatments, however, the growing use of medical resonance imaging (MRI) is allowing clinicians to chart the development of lesions. This technology is already helping scientists to evaluate new therapies. The tendency of MS to remit spontaneously leads to an array of unsubstantiated claims of cures. For example, over the years, many people have tried to implicate diet as a cause of or treatment for MS. To date, clinical studies have not been able to confirm benefits from dietary changes so patients are best advised to eat a balanced diet. Treatment strategies aim to:

- inhibit the disease process;
- promote remyelination;
- restore physical and neurological function.

Until recently, the principal treatment for MS was NSAIDs, however there is no strong evidence to support the use of these drugs to treat progressive forms of MS. Also, there is some indication that steroids may be more appropriate for people with movement, rather than sensory, symptoms. While steroids do not affect the course of MS over time, they can reduce the duration and severity of attacks in some patients.

Some potentially promising avenues of MS treatment research are:

- **Cytokines.** Synthetic forms of **IFN-β** have now been approved for use in Europe and the USA. This cytokine has been shown to reduce the number of exacerbations and may slow the progression of physical disability, with shorter and less severe attacks. In addition, **MRI** scans suggest that IFN-β can decrease myelin destruction. Alpha interferon is also being studied as a possible treatment for MS. Interleukin 4 (IL-4), an anti-inflammatory cytokine, is able to diminish demyelination and improve the clinical course of mice with EAE.

- **Immunosuppression.** The use of immunosuppressive agents can positively (if temporarily) affect the course of MS, however, toxic side-effects often preclude their widespread use. In addition, generalized immunosuppression leaves the patient open to a variety of viral, bacterial and fungal infections.

- **Myelin basic protein mimetics.** Trials of a synthetic form of MBP have shown promise in treating people in the early stages of relapsing–remitting MS. The drug appears to have few side-effects yet can reduce the relapse rate by almost one-third.

- **An MS vaccine.** Multiple sclerosis therapeutic vaccines currently under development are designed to cause the immune system to shut down the attack by autoreactive T cells on the nervous system. This would be a major treatment advance because currently available therapies are toxic and treat the individual's symptoms rather than the underlying cause of MS.

- **Peptide therapy** is based on evidence that the body can mount an immune response against the T cells that destroy myelin, but this response is not strong enough to overcome the disease. To induce this response, the TCRs of myelin-specific T cells are sequenced and a fragment, or peptide, of those receptors is then injected into the body. The immune system 'sees' the injected peptide as a foreign invader and launches an attack on any T cells that carry TCR of that specificity. Some major obstacles to developing vaccine and peptide therapies include: variation in individual patient's T cells creates a need to extract cells from each individual patient, purify the cells, and then grow them in culture before inactivating and chemically altering them. Thus the production of quantities sufficient for therapy is extremely time consuming, labour intensive, and expensive.

- **Oral tolerance.** Protein antigen feeding is similar to peptide therapy, but is a potentially simpler means to the same end. Many antigens that trigger an immune response when they are injected can lead to immunological tolerance when taken orally. Furthermore, this reaction is directed solely at the specific antigen being fed thus conferring a distinct advantage over current drug-induced immunosuppressive therapies. Data from a small, preliminary trial of antigen feeding in humans found limited suggestion of improvement, but the results were not statistically significant. It is possible that the genetics of patients, for example MHC allele expression, influences their response to oral antigen.

Sjögren's syndrome is a chronic systemic autoimmune disease. The overlapping nature of many of Sjögren's symptoms with those of other autoimmune diseases means that it is often hard to distinguish between Sjögren's and RA or systemic lupus erythematosus (SLE). The symptoms necessary for a clinical diagnosis of Sjögren's syndrome are: dry eyes, dry mouth and aching joints. In Sjögren's syndrome, the body's exocrine glands, particularly the tear glands and the salivary glands, are the targets of autoimmune attack. The glands cannot then produce the fluids that lubricate the eyes, mouth, joints and other mucosal surfaces. Other organs can be and usually are involved.

Systemic lupus erythematosus (SLE) is a chronic systemic autoimmune disease with many manifestations and affecting all of the body's organ systems. It is thought that genetic, environmental and hormonal factors play a role in its aetiology. It can occur at all ages but a younger onset is associated with a more severe course and a higher incidence of nephritis and pericarditis. It is more common in young women. The production of autoantibodies leads to immune complex formation, i.e. a Type III hypersensitivity reaction (Chapter 7). Immune complex deposition in many tissues leads to the manifestations of the disease. Immune complexes can be deposited in kidney glomeruli, skin, lungs, synovium, mesothelium, and other places. Many SLE patients develop renal complications because the immune complexes are often deposited in the renal glomeruli. A renal biopsy may be performed to determine the degree of involvement and determine therapy. Despite therapy, progression to chronic renal failure is common.

Skin rashes are common with SLE. The most characteristic rash is seen across the face, the so-called 'butterfly rash' that is accentuated by sun exposure. Systemic lupus erythematosus can be distinguished from discoid lupus erythematosus (DLE) which affects sun-exposed regions of the skin and is unlikely to be associated with systemic illness. A biopsy of sun exposed skin that is not involved with a rash will demonstrate immune complex deposition with SLE, but not with DLE.

Immune complex deposition in mesothelium can potentiate formation of effusions in body cavities. Besides pericardial effusions and serous pericarditis, SLE patients can have a form of endocarditis called Libman–Sacks endocarditis. Synovial immune complexes can lead to **arthralgias**. In fact symmetrical arthritis and arthralgias are common features such that SLE can be confused with RA early in its course. The presence of autoantibodies can usually be determined by the **antinuclear antibody (ANA)** test performed on patient serum. The titre of the ANA gives a rough indication of the severity of the disease. Not all positive ANA tests indicate autoimmune disease, particularly when the titre is low. After a positive screening ANA test, more specific tests for SLE include detection of **autoantibodies to double stranded DNA (dsDNA)**. The origin of the dsDNA is currently uncertain. Some researchers believe that it is derived from neutrophils that undergo apoptosis (programmed cell death) when skin is exposed to sunlight. The primary defect would then involve either excessive sensitivity to sunlight or a decreased ability to clear the fragments of dead neutrophils.

NSAIDs can be used, often in combination with steroids. The dose of drugs must be carefully regulated especially in patients who already have lupus nephritis (kidney damage). For people who fail conventional therapy, immunosuppressive drugs, such as cyclosporine, may be used.

Organ-specific autoimmune diseases

Acquired **autoimmune haemolytic anaemia (AIHA)** is an autoimmune disorder characterized by the premature destruction of red blood cells. Normally, the erythrocytes have a life span of approximately 120 days before they are removed by the spleen. In an individual affected with AIHA the erythrocytes are destroyed prematurely and bone marrow production of new cells can no longer compensate for their loss. The severity of this type of anaemia is determined by the time the red blood cell is allowed to survive in an affected person, and by the capacity of the bone marrow to continue red cell production.

Addison's disease (adrenal hypoplasia) is a rare disorder characterized by chronic, usually progressive, malfunctioning of the adrenal cortex. Most cases are autoimmune in origin. Deficiencies of the adrenal hormones cortisol and aldosterone result in low levels of sodium and chloride in the blood and body tissues, and high levels of potassium. Consequently, increased excretion of water and hypotension can lead to dehydration. Major symptoms of Addison's disease include fatigue, gastrointestinal discomfort, and changes in skin colour.

Autoimmune hepatitis is inflammation of the liver with consequent liver cell death. The condition is chronic and progressive although many patients present acutely ill with jaundice, fever and sometimes symptoms of severe hepatic dysfunction, a picture that resembles acute hepatitis. Autoimmune hepatitis usually occurs in women (70%) between the ages of 15 and 40. Autoimmune hepatitis should be suspected in any young patient with hepatitis, especially those without risk factors for alcohol or drug abuse, metabolic or viral disorders. Patients in whom a diagnosis of autoimmune hepatitis is suspected should have a liver biopsy. If the biopsy is consistent, treatment with steroids is begun immediately. Over the long term, many patients develop cirrhosis despite having a response to treatment, and patients who do not respond to treatment will almost always progress to cirrhosis. If end-stage liver disease develops, liver transplantation is an effective procedure. Interestingly, much of the pathology associated with autoimmune hepatitis is avoided in patients whose immune systems are compromised.

Coeliac disease is an inflammatory condition of the small intestine precipitated by the ingestion of wheat in individuals who express certain genes. The onset of illness most commonly occurs in childhood, after wheat has been introduced into the diet, and in early adult life. However it can begin at any time in life. In susceptible individuals, the wheat protein **gluten** triggers an inflammatory reaction in the small bowel which results in a decrease in the amount of surface area available for nutrient, fluid and electrolyte absorption. The mechanism by which activated inflammatory cells in the lamina propria beneath the surface epithelium of the small intestine and interspersed between epithelial cells bring about villus flattening remains a mystery. The extent of loss of intestinal absorptive surface area generally dictates whether an individual with coeliac disease will develop symptoms. Individuals with coeliac disease may experience severe symptoms such as diarrhoea, weakness and weight loss indicating a marked decrease in intestinal absorptive surface area involving much of the small intestine. The discovery of antibodies which are specific for coeliac disease, the screening of families of coeliacs and studies on selected populations have identified a growing number of asymptomatic individuals who have circulating antibodies and intestinal biopsy changes characteristic of coeliac disease. These individuals clearly have a gluten sensitivity but it is unclear whether they will develop the clinical features of coeliac disease over time. Removal of wheat (gluten) from the diet of individuals with coeliac disease or gluten sensitivity results in regeneration of the intestinal mucosal absorptive surface area and resolution of symptoms in most patients. Most patients treated with a gluten-free diet will note a lessening of symptoms within 2 weeks. There is, however, a small group of patients with presumed severe coeliac disease that is refractory to a gluten-free diet.

Gluten is a large water-insoluble protein, however the causative agent of coeliac disease has been further narrowed to smaller proline-rich proteins called **gliadins** which are capable of initiating disease in previously asymptomatic coeliacs. First-degree relatives

Some individuals with coeliac disease present with anaemia and have no symptoms that relate to the gastrointestinal tract. Such patients are likely to have disease limited to the proximal small bowel where iron is normally absorbed, with the remainder of bowel being broadly unaffected. Gluten sensitivity can also result in a blistering, burning, itchy rash on the body surface (dermatitis herpetiformis). Most of these individuals have intestinal biopsies characteristic of coeliac disease regardless of whether or not they have gastrointestinal symptoms.

of individuals with coeliac disease may or may not show symptoms of the disease. Predisposition to gluten sensitivity has been mapped to the MHC D region on chromosome 6. The most important MHC haplotype is DQw2 which is often in linkage with DR3. Other important haplotypes identified are DR7 and DPB 1, 3, 4.1 and 4.2. The sites on these MHC Class II antigens responsible for interacting with gliadin and host T cell receptors, thereby sensitizing the intestine to gluten have not been identified.

Dermatomyositis is a progressive connective tissue disorder characterized by inflammatory and degenerative changes of the muscles and of the skin. It is thought to be an autoimmune disorder although its precise origin is unknown. It involves a skin rash and muscle abnormalities that may appear together or up to a year apart. Affected individuals may experience difficulty in performing certain functions such as raising their arms and/or climbing stairs. In addition, affected individuals may experience speech and swallowing difficulties. Skin abnormalities associated with dermatomyositis typically include a reddish-purple rash on the upper eyelids (heliotrope rash); reddish-purple, horn-like growths on the surface of the knuckles, elbows, and/or knees (Grotton's sign); and/or a red rash (erythema) affecting the skin of the face, neck and/or upper torso.

Goodpasture's syndrome is a rare autoimmune disorder characterized by inflammation of the glomeruli of the kidneys (glomerulonephritis) and pulmonary haemorrhage. Symptoms of Goodpasture's syndrome include recurrent episodes of coughing up of blood (haemoptysis), difficulty in breathing (dyspnoea), fatigue, chest pain and/or anaemia. In many cases, Goodpasture's syndrome may result in acute renal failure or upper respiratory tract infection before the development of the disorder. The reason for the dual targeting of kidney and lungs is due to the sharing of epitopes on epithelial cells in these two organs.

Graves' disease is the type of hyperthyroidism caused by a generalized overactivity of the entire thyroid gland. It is also called **diffuse toxic goitre**: 'diffuse' because the entire thyroid gland is involved in the disease process; 'toxic' because the patient appears feverish as if due to an infection; and 'goitre' because the thyroid gland enlarges in this condition. The incidence of Graves' disease increases steadily throughout the first decade, with a peak during adolescence. Girls are affected 3–6 times more often than boys. Family histories are frequently positive for goitres, Graves' disease, or thyroiditis.

In Graves' disease, autoantibodies are produced against receptors on the surface of thyroid cells, stimulating those cells to over-produce thyroid hormones (Figure 8.4). The receptors normally bind thyroid-stimulating hormone (TSH), which is a regulator of the thyroid that is produced by the pituitary gland. Normal thyroid hormone production is down-regulated by a feedback loop from the circulating levels of T3 and T4, the principal thyroid hormones. The

It was the Irish physician Robert Graves who was the first to describe this form of hyperthyroidism and after whom the disease is named. Reports from the 1800s describe a mortality rate as high as 50% in patients with Graves' disease when rest and sedation were the only treatment available for the condition.

Figure 8.4 *Graves' disease is a type of hyperthyroidism caused by a generalized overactivity of the entire thyroid gland. The presence of the autoantibody against the TSH receptor overcomes the normal regulatory effect on the T3, T4 negative feedback system*

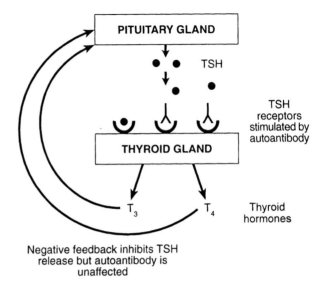

Negative feedback inhibits TSH release but autoantibody is unaffected

loop results in the shutting down of TSH production. The anti-TSH receptor antibody however is unaffected by the negative feedback and continues to stimulate the thyroid, even though TSH is absent. The main symptoms of Graves' disease are weight loss, trembling, muscle weakness of the upper arms and thighs, and insomnia. Graves' disease is the only kind of hyperthyroidism that is associated with inflammation and protrusion of the eyes. Treatment with anti-thyroid drugs, radiolabelled iodine (to be taken into the thyroid where it destroys thyroid cells) or surgery are now available and effective.

Insulin-dependent diabetes mellitus (IDDM, Type 1 diabetes) is a chronic condition in which the pancreas makes little or no insulin because the B cells in the pancreatic Islets of Langerhans have been destroyed by an autoimmune response. Insulin-dependent diabetes mellitus symptoms frequently seem to appear abruptly, although the damage to the B cells begins much earlier. The most common signs of IDDM are a great thirst, hunger, a need to urinate often, and loss of weight. To control IDDM successfully, the person must inject insulin, follow a diet plan, exercise daily, and test blood glucose several times a day. IDDM usually occurs in children and adults who are under age 40. This type of diabetes used to be known as 'juvenile diabetes', 'juvenile-onset diabetes' and 'ketosis-prone diabetes'. The most likely cure for the disease will be one that specifically blocks the immune system attack on the B cells. This would be an antigen-specific immunotherapy. It has been reported that autoimmune responses in IDDM may be primarily Th1 type. A possible way to halt the pancreatic B cell destruction would be to alter the Th1/Th2 balance in favour of Th2 responses, however the question of why a systemic Th1 response would cause the destruction only of pancreatic B cells remains unanswered.

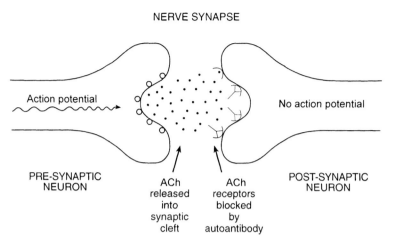

NERVE SYNAPSE

Action potential

No action potential

PRE-SYNAPTIC
NEURON

ACh
released
into
synaptic
cleft

ACh
receptors
blocked
by
autoantibody

POST-SYNAPTIC
NEURON

Figure 8.5 *The symptoms of myasthenia gravis (MG) are caused by an autoantibody that blocks acetylcholine receptors (AChR) on post-synaptic membranes in the nervous system*

Circulating autoantibodies against islet cells autoantigen (ICA) or spontaneous insulin autoantibodies (IAA) occur in some 80% of IDDM patients. IAA antibodies are not just a response to administered insulin as they may be present before treatment commences. It is important to note that IDDM patients who receive pancreatic or islet cell transplants can destroy the transplanted B cells by the same process that initiated the diabetes. Family relatives of IDDM patients possess a range of autoantibodies including ICA and IAA, indicating a pre-diabetic phase.

Myasthenia gravis (MG) is a chronic neuromuscular disease deriving its name from Latin and Greek words meaning 'grave muscle weakness'. The disease is characterized by abnormal weakness of voluntary muscles. This weakness increases with activity and decreases with periods of rest. Myasthenia gravis may affect an individual of any age or race including the newborn child, however the disease is seen more frequently in young adult females and older males. The role of heredity in MG is uncertain.

Unlike disorders such as multiple sclerosis, MG causes no progressive damage to either the nervous system or to muscles. When the disease is treated and symptoms are in remission, the MG patient can expect normal muscle function. The symptoms of MG are caused by a reduced number of acetylcholine receptors (AChRs) on post-synaptic membranes (Figure 8.5). These receptors are the normal binding site of acetylcholine (ACh), a neurotransmitter released from vesicles at the pre-synaptic membrane, during the passage of action potentials from nerves to muscles. The duration of the stimulus is limited by the enzyme acetylcholine esterase (ACh esterase) which degrades the ACh. In MG, autoantibodies are directed against many of the AChRs thereby making them unavailable to released ACh. The autoimmune response may also cause other damage to the post-synaptic membrane. The outcome is that the nervous signal cannot pass to the muscle so motor function is

Myasthenia gravis may involve either a single muscle or a group of muscles. The muscles which control chewing, swallowing and eye movement are most often affected, followed by the muscles that control the arms and legs. In some patients, the weakness is limited to ocular and eyelid muscles, resulting in double vision and/or drooping eyelids. Weakness in the muscles used for breathing may result in shortness of breath, an inability to take a deep breath, or difficulty coughing. Those MG patients who experience severe difficulty in breathing usually require hospitalization.

impaired. Continuing lack of stimulation causes the muscle to become even weaker through disuse atrophy. Testing a patient suspected of having MG involves administration of an inhibitor of ACh esterase. This prolongs the lifetime of the released ACh, thereby increasing its opportunity to bind with and stimulate the post-synaptic AChR. Patients show a transient improvement in their symptoms following drug administration.

In many adult patients the MG is accompanied by other abnormalities including thymoma (malignancy of the thymus) or thyroid hypofunction or hyperfunction. Although the disease is incurable, MG is treatable with a high degree of success.

Pernicious anaemia is a blood disorder characterized by the inability of the body to properly utilize vitamin B_{12}, which is essential for haematopoiesis. The symptoms of pernicious anaemia may include weakness, fatigue, an upset stomach, tachycardia and/or chest pains. Recurring episodes of megaloblastic anaemia and jaundice are common. Pernicious anaemia is an autoimmune disorder in which autoantibodies against **intrinsic factor**, produced by the stomach and essential for vitamin B_{12} absorption, lead to intrinsic factor destruction. Thus vitamin B_{12} cannot be absorbed. Without a cure, long-term treatment for the condition involves i.v. injection with the vitamin, i.e. bypassing the requirement for absorption. A number of rare, poorly documented late sequelae of pernicious anaemia exist, including disorders of the nervous supply to the lower limbs.

The eye may be a target of immune or inflammatory attack in many autoimmune diseases. Any autoimmune disease affecting the eye will require systemic (e.g. oral as opposed to local, topical or ocular) therapy because the components of the immune system do not reside in the eye; the eye is known as an **immunologically privileged site**. Ophthalmologists in general are not accustomed to treating patients systemically, and in particular, are not trained to use immunosuppressive drugs in order to control autoimmune phenomena. However, when the problem is identified and collaboration between ophthalmologist and other clinicians occurs it can be very effective.

Disorders of autoimmune pathogenesis occur with increased frequency in patients with previous history of another autoimmune disease. The tendency to develop another disease occurs in about 25% of these patients. Several efforts have been made to group and label these coexisting autoimmune disorders. The term **overlap syndromes** has been used to describe the group of patients that exhibit features of more than one established autoimmune disorders. For example, **mixed connective tissue disease (MCTD)** was initially described as a new syndrome with features of SLE, systemic sclerosis, polymyositis and RA and high titres of circulating antibody to nuclear ribonucleoprotein (RNP) antigen. The pathogenesis of multiple autoimmune disorders is still unknown. Multiple autoantibodies can be found in one patient and some of the specific mono- or polyclonal autoantibodies may react with multiple organs. Overall, the presence of one autoimmune disease should alert the physician to watch for a second disorder of immunological origin.

Why do autoimmune diseases occur?

With the finding of autoantibodies and autoreactive T cells in the normal circulation it can be concluded that there must exist post-thymic mechanisms that control the development of potentially damaging autoimmune reactions. Candidate mechanisms include clonal anergy, i.e. T cell clones that recognize self are maintained in a non-responsive state. Ways in which this might be achieved are through antagonistic cytokines or inhibitory TCR interactions. By analogy with proposed events in the thymus during initial T cell maturation, T cells that interact, via TCR, with an epitope require co-stimulatory signals for the response to ensue. In the absence of co-stimulators the outcome is anergy rather than response. Nonetheless, the existence of autoimmune diseases is proof that neither thymic nor post-thymic mechanisms are entirely effective.

For several decades it has been known that individuals whose cells express certain tissue types, i.e. a range of MHC antigens, have an increased risk of developing autoimmune diseases. For each disease and associated MHC antigen a relative risk (RR) may be calculated. The RR is defined as:

$$\frac{\text{Risk of a person expressing a particular MHC allele developing the disease}}{\text{Risk of a person without that MHC allele developing the disease}}$$

Table 8.1 lists the RR for a range of autoimmune diseases. These range from the strong linkage with an RR of 90 seen between ankylosing spondylitis (a degenerative rheumatoid-like muscular disorder) and allele B27 to weak linkages such as the RR of 2–4 for RA and the DW4 locus. Now that the structure and function of MHC antigens are known, we may speculate that those alleles conferring a high RR might present inappropriate epitopes, or present normal epitopes in an inappropriate manner, to T cells. Our lack of knowledge of the molecular structure of most auto-antigens makes it difficult to obtain firm confirmation of this hypothesis. Techniques for the isolation of intact MHC antigen–epitope complexes may help to resolve the problem.

The induction of self-tolerance by the thymus is thought only to involve antigen that is visible to developing T cells, i.e. present on external surfaces. Thus when previously hidden antigens are revealed they would be the target of T cell responses. Possible ways in which new antigens could appear would be through alteration of antigens or damage to cells caused by infectious agents. Other antigens might be induced to appear at a much greater concentration than previously, for example, under the

Table 8.1 *Linkage between MHC genes and risk of developing autoimmune diseases (RR = relative risk)*

Disease	MHC gene	Gene frequency in patients (%)	RR
Ankylosing spondylitis	B27	79–100	87.4
Rheumatoid arthritis	DR4	70	5.8
SLE	DR2	57	4
	DR3	46	3
Sjögren's syndrome	DR3	68–69	9.7
Type I diabetes	DW3	30–46	2.2
	DW4	48–52	4.0
Myasthenia gravis (female under 35 years)	DW3	76	12.7
Gluten sensitivity	DW3	63–93	10.8

influence of cytokines. Cell damage or cytokine expression might also increase the density of MHC Class II antigen expression on cells, so allowing antigens to be presented in concentrations likely to induce a response.

Stress proteins are a series of evolutionarily well-preserved proteins expressed in increased amounts by cells when subjected to any of a range of stresses. The best known of the stress proteins are the heat shock proteins (HSPs) and stresses that induce their synthesis include heat, hypoxia, ROS and physical trauma. One of the major functions of HSPs is to ensure correct folding of proteins within the cell. They are also thought to have a role in the peptide processing that is necessary for antigen presentation. Heat shock proteins are found in cell types from bacteria to humans. Frequently they are immunodominant. Thus, in the case of bacterial infection, the host immune system would be exposed to HSPs and would mount a response. The similarity of bacterial HSP to human HSP would then become a problem when the host produces HSP in response to any of a variety of stresses. The anti-bacterial antibodies would **cross-react** with the human HSP in an apparent autoimmune response. In RA patients, T cells have been isolated that are specific for one of the stress proteins, HSP70, which has sequence homology with both EBV glycoprotein gp110 and E. coli HSP dnaJ.

For many autoimmune diseases observations have been made that would point to an infective aetiology, however none of these hypotheses has been confirmed. Many studies have involved animals where, for example, chronic arthritis has been produced by viral infection and chronic arthritis has been transmitted to mice by a parvovirus cultured from RA synovium. A number of infectious agents have been suspected of causing MS (e.g. measles viruses), but no one particular agent has been implicated. Viral infections are usually accompanied by inflammation and the production of IFN-γ, which has been shown to worsen the clinical course of MS. It is possible that the immune response to viral infections may itself precipitate an MS attack.

The phenomenon of cross-reactivity of antibodies specific for microorganisms with host cells is known as **antigen mimicry**. A well-known example of a human disease caused by cross-reactive antibodies is rheumatic fever. This disease process begins with infection, usually a throat infection with a β-haemolytic streptococcus. Antibodies against this bacterium cross-react with myocardial cells in the heart. After some time, several years, cardiac inflammation (endocarditis) is seen. This leads to weakness of the heart muscle so the person experiences rapid fatigue and breathlessness. The best way to avoid this after-effect is to treat the initial infection rapidly with antibiotics. Thus the host immune system does not have time to mount an immune response against the organism and the infection is cleared without antibody production.

Suggested further reading

Amor, S., Baker, B., Layward, L., McCormack, K. and vanNoort, J.M. (1997) Multiple sclerosis: variations on a theme. *Immunology Today* **18**, 368–371.

Benoist, C. and Mathias, D. (1998) The pathogen connection. *Nature* **394**, 227–228.

Correale, J., Gilmore, W., Lopez, J., Li, S.Q., McMillan, M. and Weiner, L.P. (1996) Defective post-thymic tolerance mechanisms during the chronic progressive stage of multiple sclerosis. *Nature Medicine* **2**, 1354–1360.

Feldmann, M., Brennan, F.M. and Maini, R.N. (1996) Role of cytokines in rheumatoid arthritis. *Annual Review of Immunology* **14**, 397–440.

Weiner, H.L. (1997) Oral tolerance: immune mechanisms and treatment of autoimmune diseases. *Immunology Today* **19**, 335–342.

Self-assessment questions

1. Distinguish between autoimmunity and autoimmune disease.
2. What is rheumatoid factor (RF)?
3. List two clinical/laboratory findings that would allow an autoimmune disease to be distinguished from an infectious disease
4. What cytokine is considered to be of value in treating multiple sclerosis?
5. How may oral tolerance lead to antigen-specific treatments for autoimmune diseases?
6. What laboratory test is specific for the diagnosis of systemic lupus erythematosus (SLE)?

7. Explain how the autoimmune response in Graves' disease leads to over-activity of the thyroid (hyperthyroidism).
8. Relate the autoimmune response in myasthenia gravis (MG) to the observed symptoms of muscle weakness.
9. How may cellular stress in the host lead to autoimmune responses?
10. List three pieces of evidence suggesting a genetic link to the occurrence of autoimmune diseases.

Key Concepts and Facts

Autoimmune Diseases
- Autoantibodies or autoreactive T cells are thought to be causally associated with a range of different pathologies.

- Affect some 5–7% of adults in Europe and North America.

- Few autoantigens have been positively identified.

- May be organ-specific or non-organ-specific (systemic).

Non-organ Specific Autoimmune Diseases
- Involve responses to systemic autoantigens but symptoms may be confined to particular organs.

- In rheumatoid arthritis (RA), the autoantibody known as rheumatoid factor (RF) occurs in 75% of patients but its level in the serum does not always correlate with disease severity.

- The rate of occurrence of MS in identical twins is significantly less than 100% thus the disease is not entirely genetically controlled.

- Drug treatment of SLE patients must be carefully regulated as the disease process may already have caused kidney damage.

Organ-specific Autoimmune Diseases
- In pernicious anaemia autoantibodies against intrinsic factor block the absorption of vitamin B_{12}.

- Much of the pathology associated with autoimmune hepatitis does not occur in patients whose immune systems are suppressed.

- Predisposition to gluten sensitivity, that may be associated with coeliac disease, has been mapped to the MHC D region on chromosome 6.

- Circulating autoantibodies against islet cells autoantigen (ICA) or spontaneous insulin autoantibodies (IAA) occur in some 80% of patients with insulin-dependent diabetes mellitus.

Origins of Autoimmune Diseases
- Individuals whose cells express certain MHC antigens have an increased risk of developing autoimmune diseases.

- Cell damage or cytokine expression might allow the presentation of antigens not previously encountered by T cells and so lead to induction of a response.

- Anti-bacterial antibodies may cross-react with human HSP in autoimmune responses.

Chapter 9
Immune deficiency

Learning objectives

After studying this chapter you should confidently be able to:

Describe the origins of primary and secondary immune deficiencies.

Describe the consequences to the individual of impaired immune responses.

Discuss current approaches to the treatment of immune deficiencies.

The immune system is complex with multiple components and many control points. A dysfunction of any of these components or control mechanisms may lead to disordered immunity, often **immune deficiency**. Fortunately, there appears to be substantial redundancy in the immune system with some mechanisms being able to compensate for loss or dysfunction in others. Conversely, significant immune deficiencies are incompatible with life to such an extent that the affected person dies at a very young age. Modern medicine can allow people to live with previously fatal deficiencies.

Immune deficiencies involve both the natural and adaptive immune responses. They may be classified into a relatively small number of different types. Immune deficiencies may be **primary or secondary**.

Primary deficiencies are those in which the defect is within the immune system itself. These may be **congenital** (inborn) **or acquired** (appearing later in life). Any of these deficiencies may have a genetic component, however the fact that a defect is congenital does not automatically mean that it is inherited.

Secondary immune deficiencies occur as a result of a disease process or damage to some other body system which then impacts upon the mechanisms or products of the immune system.

Causes of secondary immune deficiencies include:

- ageing;
- malignancy;
- nutritional deficiencies;
- exposure to radiation;

- burns;
- immunosuppressive therapies (and other chemotherapies);
- viral infections, e.g. HIV/AIDS.

Primary immune deficiencies

Antibody deficiency syndromes may affect all antibody isotypes or only selected isotypes. The underlying defect in the disorder may be difficult to pin-point because of the dependence of B cells on T cells. Thus, when an antibody disorder is detected, it is not immediately evident whether the defect will be found in the effector population, i.e. B cells, or the in the regulatory T cell population.

X-Linked agammaglobulinaemia (XLA) was the first immunodeficiency to be identified. It is sometimes called **Bruton's disease**. It is an inherited disorder localized to the central region of the long arm of the X chromosome. The gene that is defective encodes a specific enzyme (Btk) which normally prompts B cells to become mature and able to produce antibodies. The incidence of XLA is reported to be one in 10 000.

Persons with XLA are unable to produce immunoglobulins. Most of these patients have pre B cells, but very few mature B cells. Some B cells are present in the bone marrow and circulation, but they may be reduced 100-fold or more relative to normal. Germinal centres are also absent from the lymph nodes and spleen. Patients do not have tonsils or adenoids. They are susceptible to the development of serious, pyogenic (pus producing) bacterial or viral infections. This process begins in infancy or early childhood, typically at 6–9 months of age, when the protection provided by maternally derived IgG antibodies has declined. Common infection sites are the inner ear, sinuses and respiratory tract; leading to such recurrent problems as sinusitis, conjunctivitis, otitis, rhinitis, osteomyelitis, meningitis, septicaemia, bronchitis and pneumonia. Recurrent gastrointestinal infections occur occasionally resulting in diarrhoea. Bacteria which are particularly common causes of infection in these patients include pneumococci, streptococci, staphylococci, *Pseudomonas aeruginosa* and *Hemophilus influenzae*. *Giardia lamblia* can cause gastrointestinal infections, but it is not nearly as common in XLA as in other immune deficiency diseases, e.g. common variable immunodeficiency or selective IgA deficiency.

While the cellular immunity in XLA patients is generally intact, some patients are quite susceptible to a few viruses that cause serious, life-threatening illness, for example, the viruses that cause hepatitis or poliomyelitis. Resistance to many other common infections is usually normal. Patients also tend to have an increased susceptibility to autoimmune diseases such as haemolytic anaemia and glomerulonephritis. Malignancies, including leukaemia and lymphoma, have also been reported in a few per cent of XLA patients.

Diagnosis of XLA
Measurements of the levels of immunoglobulins in the blood readily indicates deficiencies. In patients, tests have shown absences of all five immunoglobulin classes. IgG is generally less than 2 mg/mL, with IgA, IgM, IgD and IgE usually low or absent. B cell numbers may be counted and B cell function may also be assessed by measuring antibody production in response to antigen challenge. Patients do not respond to the antigen challenge.

There is no cure for XLA. Treatment with intravenous gamma-globulin needs to be sufficient to maintain serum IgG levels above 5 mg/mL in order to combat chronic infections and to prevent tissue damage. Without IgG treatment, these XLA patients may die from infections at an early age. XLA patients should not receive live viral vaccines because of the risk of developing the disease for which the vaccine was given.

Common variable immunodeficiency (CVI) is also known by other names: **hypogammaglobulinaemia, adult onset agammaglobulinaemia** or **late onset hypogammaglobulinemia**. Common variable immunodeficiency is a relatively common primary immune deficiency and affects males and females in equal numbers. The exact incidence is unknown. The disorder is characterized by a lack of antibody-producing B cells or plasma cells, low levels of most or all immunoglobulin isotypes and recurrent bacterial infections. The degree and type of deficiency, as well as its clinical signs and symptoms, vary among patients. In most patients there is a reduced amount of IgG, IgA and IgM in the blood. However, in some patients, just the IgG and IgA isotypes are reduced. B cells may be low in number and/or may fail to develop normally. Some degree of T cell dysfunction is present in up to 50% of patients.

The disorder first presents as recurrent bacterial infection in infancy and early childhood, during puberty, or even in the third, fourth or later decades of life. Because of the variable manifestations of this disorder, no clear pattern of inheritance has been observed. In most cases, there is no family history of immunodeficiency. However, in instances where more than one family member is affected, an autosomal recessive mode of inheritance is suggested.

Frequent presenting problems are recurrent infections of the ears, sinuses, bronchi and lungs. If these infections are severe and occur repeatedly permanent damage to the bronchi may occur, resulting in **bronchiectasis** (widening and scarring of the bronchial tubes). Common bacteria that often cause infection in CVI include *Hemophilus influenzae*, pneumococci and staphylococci. Gastrointestinal complaints occur frequently and may include abdominal pain, bloating, nausea, vomiting, diarrhoea or weight loss. These symptoms may be indicative of malabsorption of fat or certain sugars or may indicate the presence of the *Giardia lamblia* parasite. Gastrointestinal problems may impair normal growth and induce weight loss. In some patients whose B cells fail to develop normally, large numbers of B cells may accumulate in lymph tissue which has been stimulated by bacteria or other foreign cells. This causes marked peripheral lymph node disease and spleen enlargement. Some CVI patients develop autoantibodies against erythrocytes, leukocytes or platelets in the blood.

Treatment involves the i.v. administration of immunoglobulin concentrates. These almost always provide clinical improvement. Gammaglobulin is used but, because gammaglobulin contains little IgA or IgM, the total antibody deficiency is not replaced.

Diagnosis of CVI

When circulating immunoglobulin levels are measured in the laboratory, IgG values range from 0 to levels slightly less than normal. B cell function can be assessed by measuring antibody production after an antigenic challenge. Tests of T cell number and function can also be useful.

Selective IgA deficiency is an example of an immune deficiency in which only selected immunoglobulin isotypes are affected. This is the most common of the primary immunodeficiencies. It is defined as the total absence or severe deficiency of IgA. Blood serum levels for IgA deficient persons are usually found to be at 0.05 mg/mL or less, while serum IgA in normal adults ranges from 0.09 to 4.50 mg/mL. The disorder is termed 'selective' because other serum Ig isotypes are present at normal or increased levels. In general, selective IgA deficiency occurs once in every 400 to 2000 individuals, however its incidence varies across racial and ethnic groups. It is found most frequently in whites of European ancestry. In persons of Japanese descent, selective IgA deficiency occurs in only 1 in 18 500 persons.

IgA is deficient in patients because their B cells are unable to make the isotype switch necessary to become IgA-producing plasma cells. Thus, IgA deficient persons have IgA-bearing B cells that are arrested at an immature stage of development. The lack or severe deficiency of IgA at its usual body sites, i.e. mucosal surfaces, causes increased susceptibility to recurrent infection, allergies, chronic diarrhoea or autoimmune diseases. The functions of T cells, phagocytes and complement are normal or near-normal.

The exact cause or causes of selective IgA deficiency has not yet been determined although there is evidence of familial inheritance. Selective IgA deficiency also occurs frequently in immediate relatives of persons with CVI, suggesting a similar cause for the two disorders. In rare cases, partial IgA deficiency has been linked variously to deletions of the IgA1 or IgA2 genes on chromosome 14, to MHC genes on chromosome 6 or to partial deletion of the long or short arm of chromosome 18. Nonetheless the vast majority of persons with selective IgA deficiency have no evidence of chromosomal abnormalities.

IgA-deficient persons may vary from being healthy and symptom-free to having significant illness. Thus, some IgA-deficient persons may be totally unaware of their antibody deficiency with no more than the usual number of upper respiratory infections and/or occasional diarrhoea. The reason why some IgA-deficient persons have more illness than others is not clear, however some patients become ill during infancy while others may be healthy into their 60s and 70s. IgA deficiency does not become detectable until approximately 6 months of age. For those IgA-deficient patients with a history of recurrent infections, the most common problems are ear infections, sinusitis and pneumonia. Other infection sites can be the throat, gastrointestinal tract or eyes. These infections may become chronic and may not completely clear up with a course of antibiotics, necessitating prolonged antibiotic therapy. Some IgA-deficient people with significant illness may also be missing a fraction of their IgG (IgG2) antibodies.

Allergies, usually asthma and food allergies, are another common problem with selective IgA deficiency and these may range from

The association of mental retardation with IgA deficiency has been found in patients with ataxia–telangiectasia, a hereditary, progressive disease. Additionally, Selective IgA deficiency can occur as a consequence of congenital intrauterine infection with rubella (German measles); toxoplasmosis (a disease caused by protozoan infection); or cytomegalovirus (CMV).

mild to severe. A more unusual form of allergy that occurs in persons who have a total absence of IgA is an allergic reaction to IgA. Exposure through blood products containing IgA causes some IgA deficient individuals to develop antibodies against this foreign protein. In some cases this antibody may develop spontaneously, without exposure to IgA. Administration of blood products to IgA-deficient patients may induce anaphylactic shock. If an IgA-deficient person is tested and found to carry anti-IgA antibodies, they should receive washed red blood cells, or blood products, from an IgA-deficient donor or from autologous blood donation.

Autoantibodies may be present in some 40% of cases of IgA deficiency. These autoantibodies are directed against many auto-antigens including: IgG, smooth muscle, mitochondria, basement membrane and thyroglobulin (a protein from the thyroid gland). The presence of such antibodies is not necessarily associated with disease, however autoimmune diseases are a common clinical presentation of persons with selective IgA deficiency. The auto-immune diseases most frequently seen in selective IgA deficiency are RA, SLE, Sjögren's syndrome, thyroiditis, haemolytic anaemia and chronic active hepatitis.

There is no cure or effective treatment for selective IgA deficiency. Any treatment is directed toward the specific disease associated with the deficiency, if any. Gammaglobulin treatment is not used in IgA deficiency unless IgG deficiency is also present. Commercial gam-maglobulin preparations do not contain much IgA, and even if IgA-rich preparations were produced, the infused IgA would not go to the mucous membranes where this protein is needed.

In **Immunodeficiency with Hyper IgM** (also called **hyper-IgM syndrome**) serum IgA and IgG are severely deficient, whereas IgM is elevated. The clinical course is like that of XLA except for a greater frequency of 'autoimmune' haematological disorders (neutropae-nia, haemolytic anaemia, thrombocytopaenia). In contrast to XLA patients who lack tonsils, tonsillar hypertrophy may occur in hyper-IgM patients due to infiltration with IgM-containing plasma cells. Neutropaenia may also be present leading to gingivitis, ulcerative stomatitis, fever and weight loss. The disorder appears to involve a primary dysfunction of the B cell isotype switching from IgM to IgG and IgA. The disorder is X-linked recessive; female carriers have normal IgG and IgA.

Some recent work has led to a greater understanding of the possible defect in this condition. Patients with hyper-IgM express functional CD40 but their T cells do not have functional ligand for CD40 (CD40L). The CD40L gene locus corresponds to the site where the clinical phenotype of the hyper-IgM syndrome had been mapped. There is now conclusive evidence that the defect in X-linked hyper-IgM syndrome resides in the CD40L gene. Point mutations in this gene have been found in 75% of patients with the syndrome. Activated T cells from affected patients fail to express wild-type CD40L, although their B cells may respond

---

Diagnosis of selective IgA deficiency

IgA levels in the blood or serum may be measured by single radial diffusion, radioimmunoassay, ELISA or automated laser nephelometry. In the IgA-deficient patient, IgA levels will either be absent or below 0.05 mg/mL, while other isotypes are normal. In a small percentage of cases, perhaps 10%, an IgA-deficient patient may also be deficient in IgG2. T cells, phagocytic cells and the complement system are normal or near normal. Other tests, e.g. for autoantibodies, would depend on the patient's symptoms.

normally to wild-type CD40L. Patients with the hyper-IgM syndrome do not express IgE, strongly indicating that CD40L is required (in conjunction with IL-4) for production of IgE *in vivo*.

The demonstration of mutations in the T cell producing CD40L is consistent with the suspicion of a primary T cell defect because of the recurrence of opportunistic infections (Pneumocystis carinii pneumonia, toxoplasmosis) generally associated with anomalies of T cell function. This defect emphasizes the central role of the CD40L/CD40 interaction in immunoglobulin class switching.

IgG subclass deficiency occurs when there is an imbalance of the IgG subclasses with one or more subclasses being deficient. The overall level of IgG can be normal, but individual subclass levels may be higher or lower than normal. The incidence of this fairly common primary immune disorder is not yet known. In most cases affected individuals have increased susceptibility to infection and have a history of frequent pyogenic infections since childhood, low or normal serum Ig levels, and selective deficiencies of IgG subclasses 1, 2, 3 or 4. Some people with IgG subclass deficiency are perfectly healthy. Patients usually present with a history of frequent infections involving the respiratory tract such as otitis media (ear infection); sinusitis; bronchitis and pneumonia. The causes of these infections are often found to be encapsulated bacteria such as *Hemophilus influenzae* and *Streptococcus pneumoniae*, especially in the case of an IgG2 deficiency. Lung function impairment and bronchiectasis also have been reported in these patients. Some patients develop autoimmunity. IgG2 deficient patients may have a poor response to some vaccines, such as pneumococcal, or *Hemophilus influenzae* vaccines. The levels of IgG subclasses in children are not always stable over time. They may change with age or may normalize. Also, the sex distribution among children affected with this disorder may change as time passes. The subclass of IgG deficiency has also been seen to change with time, with IgG2 deficiency predominant in children and IgG3 deficiency predominant in adults.

The cause of IgG subclass deficiency is unknown. It may be associated with IgA deficiency and may be more common in families in which CVI is found. Administration of i.v. gammaglobulin has been shown in some studies to reduce the number of infections in patients and so reduce their dependence on antibiotics.

Not all immune deficiencies are irreversible. In fact, many children may experience **transient immune deficiency due to hypogammaglobulinaemia** that reverses as soon as the child's immune system becomes sufficiently mature to generate its own Ig. Figure 9.1 illustrates the sources of Ig within the child during pregnancy and the first two years of life. It can be seen that the last trimester is critical for the transfer of maternal IgG to the foetus. This is augmented by IgA that is present in the mother's milk, especially in colostrum, the first milk produced. In the normal healthy child this maternal Ig is sufficient to provide protection until the baby's Ig

The CD40 molecule is a glycoprotein expressed on B cells, epithelial cells and some cancer cells. Cross-linking of CD40 by anti-CD40 monoclonal antibodies mediates B cell proliferation, adhesion and differentiation. The human CD40 (CD40L) ligand can be detected on T cells but is absent from B cells and monocytes. It is expressed on both CD4$^+$ and CD8$^+$ T cells. IL-4, an inducer of IgE production, upregulates CD40L mRNA levels while IFN-γ, an inhibitor of IgE synthesis, reduces expression of CD40L mRNA. Thus there appears to be a correlation between human CD40L expression and IgE production.

The methods of choice for diagnosing IgG subclass deficiency are radial immunodiffusion, ELISA, RIA or other methods. Test results also vary from one laboratory to another despite careful control of reagents and methodology. No uniform methods are established and deficiency of a given subclass may not correlate with clinical disease. A most important indicator is the determination of the response to vaccines; if a person with an IgG2 subclass defect has a poor response to pneumococcal vaccine, a true antibody defect is present. One problem is that IgG subclass values may vary from laboratory to laboratory. Various minor abnormalities of B cell and T cell levels and function also have been reported.

Figure 9.1 *The development of Ig synthesis in the newborn takes place over a period of 2 years. Protection by maternal Ig is critical and lasts for several months after birth*

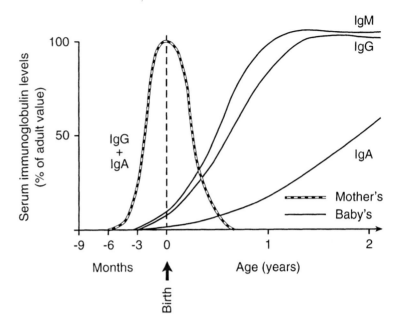

levels are raised. Babies that are born prematurely usually miss a lot of the transfer of maternal IgG and, because they frequently have difficulties in breastfeeding, they fail to receive IgA. Commercial baby milk formulae do not contain human antibodies. The lowered resistance to infection found in premature babies, e.g. because of deficiency in lung surfactant that normally aids the removal of microorganisms from the lungs, is thus exacerbated by lowered antibody-mediated immunity.

Deficiencies of cell-mediated immunity

All components of the immune system are subject to deficiencies, including cell-mediated immunity. Instead of a long list of T cell deficiencies, however, there are relatively few. One reason for this may be that impairment of the T cell system is incompatible with life. Three T cell deficiencies that have been recognized are DiGeorge's syndrome, Wiskott–Aldrich syndrome and Nezelof syndrome.

DiGeorge's syndrome, also called **thymic aplasia** (failure of the thymus to develop naturally) or **thymic hypoplasia** (defective development of thymic tissue) is a congenital immune disorder characterized by lack of embryonic development or underdevelopment of the pharyngeal pouches. The syndrome is often associated with congenital heart defects, anomalies of blood vessels, oesophageal atresia (congenital failure of oesophageal tube to develop), abnormalities of facial structures and low levels of serum calcium as a result of the hypoparathyroidism (insufficient activity of the parathyroid glands). In most cases there is a defect on chromosome

22. Depending on the degree of parathyroid or thymic hypoplasia, hypocalcaemic tetany (intermittent spasms of the extremities) may be present. Regardless of the form or severity of involvement, most patients are recognized clinically by characteristic external features that include:

- abnormally increased distance between eyes;
- low-set, prominent ears;
- unusual smallness of the jaws and mouth without the usual bow-shape of the upper lip.

Several cardiac abnormalities are also associated with DiGeorge's syndrome. The immunological defects in patients are, in fact, quite variable and spontaneous remissions have been reported. These children also have depressed antibody response to specific antigens and, in older patients, defective primary and secondary antibody responses to multiple agents also are noted. The occurrence of DiGeorge's syndrome is sporadic. Most patients have a partial defect and will, over time, become normal or nearly normal immunologically. The best treatment of the immune defects of DiGeorge's syndrome is controversial. Whether transplant with foetal thymus (thymus of 10–15-week-old stillborn foetus) works or not is debated.

Wiskott–Aldrich syndrome (WAS) is manifested as eczema, thrombocytopaenia, proneness to infection and bloody diarrhoea. The thrombocytopaenia in people with the disorder is accompanied by elevated platelet-associated IgG and low mean platelet size. Both return to normal after splenectomy. Patients who relapse redevelop elevated IgG but maintain normal platelet size. However death usually occurs before the age of 10 years. There is evidence that the immune defect is one of antigen processing or recognition, perhaps due to abnormalities in the cytoskeleton of leukocytes. The incidence of WAS is 4.0 per million live male births in the USA. Causes of death are mainly infections or bleeding but some 10% of patients develop malignancies, usually leukaemias.

Nezelof's syndrome (NS) involves T cell deficiency with little or no abnormality of Ig; the defect may be limited to the thymus. Impaired delayed hypersensitivity occurs and there are no skin reactions to such stimuli as mumps. Skin grafts are not rejected. Patients with NS tend to succumb in early childhood to infections. Humoral immunity is near-normal but despite normal or increased levels of one or more of the major Ig classes, antibody synthesis is impaired. Family studies suggest an autosomal recessive inheritance.

Combined deficiencies of antibody-mediated and cell-mediated immunity

Some of the most serious immune deficiencies seen are those in which both B cells and T cells appear to be affected. The principal type is **severe combined immune deficiency (SCID)**. Severe combined immune deficiency results in marked susceptibility to severe and complicated infections. The onset of infection usually occurs in the first 6 months of life. It is considered to be the most serious of the primary immune disorders. The exact incidence of SCID is unknown, but it is rare in most population groups, probably of the order of 1 in 1 000 000. Severe combined immune deficiency is actually a group of disorders. The most common forms are either X-linked or autosomal recessive. This immune disorder arises most commonly as either a genetic mutation isolated to the proximal part of the long arm of the X chromosome, an inherited autosomal recessive disorder or a deficiency of the enzyme adenosine deaminase (ADA). Approximately 30% of children diagnosed with SCID are ADA deficient.

The main features of SCID are:

- T cells function poorly or are absent;
- the thymus may be small and functions poorly or is absent;
- bone marrow stem cells, from which T cells and B cells arise, are absent or defective;
- there is little or no antibody production.

Stem cells in the bone marrow are defective or absent. With the absence or poor function of T cells and/or thymus, the normal functioning of both T and B cells is impaired. While it is not known exactly why these defects occur, it is believed that the defect or error occurs during foetal development.

In cases of **ADA deficiency**, immunodeficiency occurs because of a build up of metabolic substrates in the lymphocytes. These children may present at a slightly older age because, in many cases, the deficiency is mild and it takes time for the metabolic substrates to accumulate. This is an autosomal recessive form of SCID.

SCID infants present with an unusual number of bacterial, viral, fungal or protozoal infections that are much more life-threatening, serious, and non-responsive to treatment than would normally be expected. These include, but are not limited to, pneumonia, meningitis and/or septicaemia. Haematological abnormalities are common and may include neutropaenia, anaemia, eosinophilia and monocytosis. The increased leukocyte numbers may signal the presence of infections such as *Pneumocystis carinii* pneumonia. These patients can have a large liver and/or spleen, or palpable or enlarged lymph nodes.

Exposure to the chicken pox virus, either through live vaccine or in the environment, can be life-threatening with infection of the lungs and/or brain. The relatively common and harmless cytomegalovirus (CMV), found in the salivary glands of many people, can cause fatal pneumonia in children with SCID. Even the herpes simplex virus (which causes the common cold sore) and the measles

Pending correction of the immune defect, children with SCID should be isolated from children outside the family and even their own brothers and sisters as the latter are likely to be exposed to viruses (especially chicken pox), bacteria or fungi. Siblings should be vaccinated with only killed virus because they may continue to excrete live virus, which could be dangerous to the immune compromised patient. The patients should never receive live virus vaccines. Other precautions include hand washing, good nutrition (which may include intravenous feeding) and prophylactic doses of antibiotics. Although it does not replace B cell deficiency, gammaglobulin therapy can be used to restore antibody levels in the blood until the B cell system is restored by transplantation.

virus can be dangerous to these children. Fungal infections such as mouth thrush (*Candida albicans*) and a yeast infection in the nappy area may be resistant to treatment that would be effective for someone with a normal immune system. Persistent diarrhoea is common in these patients and may lead to severe weight loss and malnutrition. Other gastrointestinal problems include chronic hepatitis or bile duct damage. Skin problems may persist, including chronic skin infections and fungal infections.

The treatment of choice for children with SCID is bone marrow transplantation, ideally from a normal sibling donor. The ideal donor is matched at the MHC HLA-A, HLA-B and HLA-D loci, with HLA-D being the most important match to ensure significant survival. Prior to transplantation, the patient undergoes irradiation or immunosuppressive chemotherapy to eliminate host bone marrow stem cells that may be deficient. Any mature T or B cells in the bone marrow should be removed as these cells would contribute to graft-versus-host disease. In the absence of a tissue-matched sibling, patients can be given a T cell depleted bone marrow transplant from a relative or other partially matched donor. Restoration of cellular immunity occurs 3–6 months following successful transplantation while normal antibody production may take 1–3 years. During this period, gammaglobulin therapy should be used to provide protection against recurrent pyogenic infections. Recent success rates for this procedure approach 80% for matched bone marrow donors. Without a bone marrow transplant, a child with SCID is at constant risk of severe or fatal infection and may be best kept in sterile isolation. Without treatment, survival beyond the first year of life is unusual.

The **bare lymphocyte syndrome (BLS)** is a member of the relatively heterogeneous class of SCID. It is associated with, and probably results from, the lack of expression of MHC antigens on some cells of haematopoietic origin. Both MHC Class I and Class II antigens may be affected. In addition to being of interest in its own right as a 'cause' of SCID, BLS provides insight into the role of MHC antigens in lymphocyte differentiation and validates the role of MHC antigens in normal immune responses. The affected children can be of both sexes with first symptoms presenting after the age of 3 or 4 months. Death due to chronic diarrhoea and repeated bacterial and viral infections frequently occurs in childhood. It is possible that the numbers of T and B cells are normal yet functions of both cell types are absent. Successful bone marrow transplantations can be carried out although the determination of patient MHC haplotype is made very difficult because of the non-expression of the genes on lymphocytes.

The laboratory diagnosis of SCID involves both quantitative and qualitative tests including lymphocyte counting, lymphocyte function tests, and evaluation of levels of IgG, IgA and IgM. Results of all of these tests will be decreased in SCID patients compared with normal. It is important to rule out the possibility that such results are due to the presence of viral infections. Tests which identify carriers allow prenatal diagnosis in some families in which the X-linked form of SCID has been previously identified. However, as with all X-linked disorders, more than half of affected males represent the first manifestation of a new mutation in their families.

Deficiencies of non-specific immunity

Deficiencies of complement components may lead to increased frequency of infections, particularly bacterial. Deficiency of factor

C3 is the most severe as it is normally present in the highest concentration and contributes to activation through both the classical and alternate pathways. Deficiencies in components C5, C6, C7, C8 or C9 still permit formation of the membrane attack complex although it will be slightly less efficient than normal. Deficiencies in complement inhibitors may lead to inappropriate complement activation. This wastage of complement can cause a deficient response during infections when increased complement activation is required.

The features of **Chediak–Higashi syndrome (CHS)** are decreased pigmentation of hair and eyes (partial albinism), photophobia, nystagmus, large eosinophilic, peroxidase-positive inclusion bodies in the myeloblasts and promyelocytes of the bone marrow, neutropaenia, abnormal susceptibility to infection, and malignant lymphoma. Death often occurs before the age of 7 years. Large lysosomal granules occur in leukocytes with giant melanosomes in melanocytes. Neutrophils show deficient chemotaxis and bactericidal activities. Deficiencies of lysosomal enzymes in these cells may account for the impaired bacterial killing. Defects of natural killer (NK) cells are also present that may have some link with the development of malignancy in CHS patients.

Chronic granulomatous disease (CGD) is an inherited disorder characterized by neutrophils which are unable to kill certain microorganisms. Chronic granulomatous disease occurs once in every 1 million persons. It is more common in males than females, by a ratio of 4 to 1. Approximately 80% of patients develop the disease through an X-linked form of inheritance, while about 20% inherit through an autosomal recessive pattern.

In CGD patients, neutrophils move normally to the site of a microbial invasion and even ingest the microorganism however, after ingestion, killing of the phagocytosed organism(s) cannot take place. The reason for this is that a respiratory burst does not occur due to absence, or defect, of the enzyme NADPH oxidase. Patients with CGD have an increased susceptibility to recurrent, serious infections by bacteria and fungi. These infections usually involve the skin, soft tissues, respiratory tract, lymph nodes, liver, spleen or bones. To clear these infections may require prolonged antibiotic treatment.

Fewer than 30% of children with CGD have infectious problems before 3 months of age. However, problems begin to surface soon after, with about 80% developing unusually frequent or severe infections before age 2. In most cases, these infections lead to formation of granulomas (Chapter 8). Granulomas may involve any part of the body, but usually are found in the skin, lungs, lymph nodes, liver or bones. Occasionally granulomas may cause obstructions of the intestine or urinary tract. Ultimately, these lesions may remain for a long period of time after treatment, heal slowly and may leave residual scarring. Recurrent problems for these patients

---

Diagnosis of CGD

Leukocytosis is likely to be present, secondary to an increase of juvenile and segmented neutrophils. There is also likely to be anaemia; elevated ESR and hypergammaglobulinaemia in which IgG, IgM and IgA are elevated. IgE levels may be increased. Skin tests for delayed hypersensitivity are positive. Specific diagnostic tests of leukocyte function are likely to show decreased Nitroblue Tetrazolium (NBT) reduction and decreased chemiluminescence; both due to the lack of oxygen reduction reactions in affected neutrophils. Direct measurements of superoxide anion production will also show defects. *Staphylococcus aureus, Staphylococcus epidermidis, Serratia marcescens, Escherichia coli* and *Aspergillus* are the most common microorganisms recovered from infection sites.

include pneumonia, lung abscesses, and other chronic lung infections.

There is no specific corrective therapy for patients with CGD although early bone marrow transplantation has been done in a few cases. Gamma interferon is now a standard treatment. This cytokine works in a number of ways to reduce the number of infections these patients develop, including increasing the expression of NADPH oxidase by neutrophils. The side-effects of IFN-γ include fever, muscle aches and fatigue. Newer approaches being investigated include the possibility of using gene therapy to restore the missing normal NADPH oxidase genes into patients cells.

In **leukocyte adhesion deficiency (LAD)** some of the adhesion molecules that normally permit leukocytes to migrate to the site of infection may be absent. Those most likely to be affected are the β-integrins.

Secondary immune deficiencies

Immunosuppressive drugs: following transplantation of tissues or organs, generally known as **grafts**, it is necessary to minimize the risk of rejection responses developing in the recipient. This requires that their immune responses be suppressed using drugs. There are two basic suppression strategies:

- non-antigen specific (generalized);
- antigen specific.

Generalized immunosuppression is by far the more frequently employed. The drugs used suppress all responses. The most common are:

- **Corticosteroids**. These have well-known anti-inflammatory properties but also significant side-effects through prolonged or high dose usage.
- Drugs that target rapidly proliferating cells, e.g. lymphocytes proliferating in response to an antigenic stimulus. The drugs currently used include methotrexate, cyclophosphamide and azathioprine. Their side-effects include the destruction of other rapidly proliferating cells such as those lining the gut. The same drugs are also used in some regimens for chemotherapy of cancer, i.e. another situation where drugs are used to target rapidly proliferating cells. Thus cancer chemotherapy may lead also to secondary immune deficiencies. The management of patients undergoing chemotherapy usually involves allowing them sufficient time between doses of drugs for their leukocyte numbers to recover and hence to minimize the complication of diminished resistance to infection.

- Cyclosporin A. This drug, which was originally isolated from a fungus, inhibits T cell proliferation by interfering with IL-2 synthesis. Some recent evidence indicates that its prolonged use may lead to the development of certain cancers.
- Other bacterial-derived molecules, e.g. **FK506 and rapamycin.**
- Antibodies that interfere with, or destroy, T cells, e.g. **OKT3 or anti-lymphocyte globulin (ALG).**
- **X-irradiation** to destroy the recipient's leukocytes. (Inadvertent exposure to radiation causes profound immune deficiency.)

One important side-effect of all of these treatments is that they predispose the patient to infections of all types with potentially serious consequences. Most transplant recipients need to take some level of immunosuppression for the whole of their lives. The balance between risk of rejection and risk from infectious disease is one that must be maintained through constant vigilance and clinical follow-up, i.e. if there are signs of infection, the dose of immunosuppressive drug is reduced until it is cleared. If there is any sign of rejection, the dose is raised. One way to overcome this problem is to develop effective **antigen-specific immunosuppressive therapies.** Antigen-specific mechanisms would allow the inhibition only of those responses targeted on the graft; all responses against other antigens could proceed as normal. Currently, this type of immunosuppression involves procedures that manipulate specific aspects of responses, rather than individual drugs. Some such procedures are:

- **Destruction of 'passenger' lymphocytes** within the graft prior to transplantation. This can be done using specific antibodies to T cells.
- **Multiple blood transfusions.** The potential recipient receives several blood transfusions from the donor. This causes a reduction in the extent of responses directed against donor cells.

For many years it was hypothesized that people developed **malignant tumours** because they had a deficiency in immune responses that normally destroyed cancer cells as they arose. Real evidence for such a deficiency was not forthcoming, however, even though a wide range of impaired responses can be measured in patients with cancer. Whether the deficiencies led to or resulted from the disease could not be deduced from such observations and, further, the wide range of metabolic disturbances, some resulting from treatment, that are present in cancer patients could underlie impaired responsiveness. Data obtained from animal, usually murine, models of cancers were often misleading primarily because most human cancers arise spontaneously whereas animal tumours were induced by direct chemical action or the transplantation of tumour cells. Strong anti-tumour immune responses could be observed in animals. However most human cancers are now known to induce only very weak responses. One reason for this is because tumour cells arise from the host, and hence strongly resemble the normal self cells. A role for immune deficiency in the development of human cancer cannot be substantiated.

Older people are afflicted by a large variety of infectious problems, which are accompanied by higher mortality rates than those seen in the younger population. The increase in some infections is dramatic, such as the strong association of herpes zoster with increasing age. Others are more subtle, such as the increased risk of mortality due to influenza in the elderly. Many factors can contribute to this phenomenon, including a reduced ability to mount protective immune responses (**immunosenescence**) (Table 9.1).

Physical barriers against non-self decline with age: there is thinning and drying of the skin and a decline in its blood flow and the mucous membranes become drier and more susceptible to injury or invasion by bacteria. Chemotaxis and ingestion of organisms appear to be normal but, once organisms are ingested, elderly individuals' neutrophils are less able to kill microbes.

Thymic wasting, or involution accompanies ageing and may give a clue to the immune dysfunction that accompanies old age. In some studies, administration of thymic hormones or grafting of thymic tissue can reverse some of the immune age-related deficits. Other immunological sites in the body, e.g. GALT, do not appear to decline with age so they may provide avenues to circumvent the immunodeficiency. The number of B cells changes little in older humans but, in contrast, the changes in T cell and NK subtypes in the elderly are quite dramatic. The number of mature $CD8^+$ T cells declines with age while $CD4^+$ T cells show little change in absolute

Table 9.1 *Immune changes associated with ageing*

Immune function	Alteration
Innate immunity	Skin/mucous membranes thinned, dry, mild decrease in blood flow
Complement	Normal
Chemotaxis	Normal
Ingestion	Normal
Intracellular killing	Decreased
T cell development in thymus	Decreased
T cell development in GALT	Normal
T cell/B cell subpopulations	Shift to activated/memory cells
NK cells	Increased
Lymphocyte proliferation	Decreased
IL-1 expression/secretion	Normal
IL-2, IL-2 receptor, IL-12	Decreased
IL-4, IL-6, IL-10, IFN-γ	Increased
Delayed-type hypersensitivity	Decreased

number. There is also a shift from naive T cell subpopulations to those associated with activated or memory T cells in mouse and human studies. This shift may influence cytokine production.

Since lymphocyte subpopulations may also shift in response to illness, some of the published data on lymphocyte subsets in the aged may be confounded by these concomitant pathologies. The SENIEUR protocol, a longitudinal, observational cohort study of healthy elderly, was one attempt to determine which changes are specifically due to ageing rather than to comorbid conditions. Investigators in the SENIEUR study found virtually no differences in the number of circulating $CD3^+$ or $CD4^+$ T lymphocytes and only a slight decline in $CD8^+$ T lymphocytes in older people. However, these investigators found marked elevations in the number of circulating NK cells. This difference was even greater in subjects who demonstrated some evidence of malnutrition, (albumin <35 mg/mL), despite being clinically healthy. **Nutritional abnormalities** are common in the elderly and may compound immunosenescence. Undernourished elders are more likely than their well-nourished counterparts to die from infectious diseases. Even modest systemic nutritional deficiency results in a decline of delayed-type hypersensitivity (DTH) responses and a decreased number of total and mature T cells. Neutrophil function is reduced, and while phagocytosis is generally not affected, the ability to destroy ingested bacteria appears to decline.

The most prominent change in immune function associated with ageing is the change in lymphocyte proliferative responses. Lymphocyte proliferative responses gradually decline throughout life. The decrease in proliferative responses may be due to a decline in expression of IL-2 receptors. Paradoxically, lymphocyte responses may not be decreased in the 'oldest' elderly population (i.e. >90 years), possibly reflecting a strong survivor bias that may be linked to specific genotypes.

Changes in cytokine production may compromise cell-mediated immunity in the elderly. The cytokine profile may change to generally favour the production of antibodies, rather than cellular immunity. Enhanced IL-10 secretion from non-T cell sources has been linked to autoantibodies, a common finding in the elderly. Skin testing with a panel of common antigens to which most individuals have become immune throughout life is a good measure of how well their immune system is responding. Unresponsiveness to antigens to which they were previously exposed is common in subjects over 65 years of age.

Infectious diseases may be a serious complication in patients who have sustained serious burns. The principal reason for this is that they may have lost significant amounts of skin, the major barrier against invasion of non-self. Patients who have inhaled smoke/heat may also have damage to the mucus membranes of the lungs. The immune systems of patients may function normally however non-cellular components, antibodies, cytokines, acute phase proteins etc, may also be lost due to the persistent loss of extracellular fluids that occurs until an effective skin barrier is re-established.

HIV infection and acquired immune deficiency syndrome (AIDS)

In the late 1970s and early 1980s young people, predominantly men, were seen to be presenting to hospitals and clinics in the USA with symptoms of infectious disease not normally seen in people of their age group in westernized countries. Intensive research into their condition, and the as-yet incomplete search for a cure, has been by far the most significant reason for the increased understanding of immunology that has emerged over the past decade or so. The underlying defect that led to their symptoms was an immune deficiency resulting from infection with the virus now known as **human immune deficiency virus (HIV)**. The immune deficiency is **acquired immune deficiency syndrome (AIDS)**.

AIDS is a worldwide problem, with most cases occurring in sub-Saharan Africa, Asia (primarily India), South America and the USA. It is transmitted when blood or blood products are exchanged through:

- sexual intercourse;
- blood transfusions;
- sharing of apparatus for intravenous drug use or injections;
- trans-placental transfer during pregnancy or lactation.

HIV is a retrovirus, i.e. it carries RNA as its genetic material. As an obligate parasite, the HIV can replicate only within nucleated cells. Viruses do not invade host cells randomly but do so through interaction with specific receptors. **The receptor for HIV is the CD4 molecule** that occurs in highest density on $CD4^+$ T cell but also on macrophages and macrophage-like cell throughout the body, e.g. glial cells and astrocytes in the brain and CNS, dendritic cells in lymph nodes, etc. Some years ago it was recognized that CD4 alone on a cell surface is insufficient to allow infection by HIV; a co-receptor is necessary. The co-receptors are now known to be receptors for chemokines (similar to cytokines) that are known as **CXCR4 and CCR5** (Figure 9.2). Once it has infected the $CD4^+$ cell the HIV must transcribe its RNA into DNA. This step is catalysed by the enzyme **reverse transcriptase** and it permits the subsequent integration of HIV genes into the host genome. Transcription of host genes will also cause transcription of HIV genes leading to the formation of new viral particles. It is an interesting fact that the fate of all $CD4^+$ cells that become infected with HIV may not be the same. The observed immune deficiency results from the destruction of $CD4^+$ T cells. Other $CD4^+$ cells probably are not destroyed at anything like the same rates as the T cells although $CD8^+$ cell death contributes to the exhaustion of the

Figure 9.2 *Infection of CD4⁺ cells by HIV involves interaction of CD4 molecules with gp120 and gp41 on the virus surface*

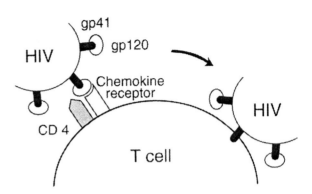

Anti-HIV antibodies provide the basis of the most frequently used test for exposure to HIV. There are several targets for the antibodies, including gp120 on the envelope and the core protein p24. The techniques used are ELISA, western blotting and PCR.

immune system and killing of neurons in the brain leads to dementia.

In the early stages of the infection a vigorous immune response is mounted. This is apparent in the production of antibodies against the free (extracellular) virus. Antibodies contribute to the removal of virus from extracellular environments, however much of the virus rapidly enters CD4⁺ cells so **antibody-mediated responses are ineffective**. Further, the antibodies may actually enhance HIV invasion into cells through interaction of HIV:antibody complexes with Fc receptors. The intracellular viruses begin to multiply rapidly and are released from host cells. This phase is detectable by the high levels of virus particles in the blood. Cytotoxic T cell (CTL) responses are also activated and there is destruction of HIV-infected cells. This is the principal mechanism through which the number of CD4⁺ T cells decreases. The reduction in the viral load that is brought about by these early immune responses allows the infection to enter its **latent phase**.

The latent phase should not be considered as a stage when virus remains 'hidden' in CD4⁺ cells, ignored by the immune system. Rather the latent phase appears to involve constant skirmishes between virus and CTLs. The HIV continues to replicate, mostly in secondary lymphoid tissues, for example lymph nodes, and CTL activity is induced in response. For long periods (typically 5–10 years) this continues and the immune system seems to have sufficient resources to cope with the high level of T cell death and consequent need for replacement. Nonetheless, a point is reached where the relentless reproductive capacity of the virus allows it to gain supremacy over the immune system that has been weakened in a number of important ways:

- Many of the **T cells that are destroyed are memory cells** hence the ability of the infected person to respond to previously encountered antigen is reduced.

- The **persistent CTL** responses in the lymphoid tissues cause damage to those tissues and hence they are unable to support the normal proliferative and differentiation activity of the B and T cells which they contain.

- The bone marrow produces new cells that will become lympho-cytes, however our current state of knowledge would suggest that the level of regulation of this activity is insufficient to favour the production of the necessary $CD4^+$ T cells over other lymphocyte types for which there is not so great a need. Further new evidence indicates that HIV may be able to inhibit the ability of the bone marrow to produce leukocytes.

Throughout the years of latency, the HIV is never totally destroyed by the immune response. The principal reason for this is that $CD4^+$ cells other than T cells, e.g. macrophages, persist in the tissues as reservoirs of virus. Any stimulus that causes the activation or destruction of these cells, e.g. other infectious agents, will cause the release of large numbers of virus particles into the circulation.

Towards the end of the latent period the ability of the immune system to deal effectively with HIV declines. The rate of decline becomes particularly steep as the patient enters the final stages of the disease. This stage is known as AIDS and it can be defined by both laboratory and clinical criteria (Table 9.2). Patients usually die from multiple, overwhelming infection with opportunistic patho-gens, i.e. organisms that would not cause significant illness in healthy hosts and a skin cancer known as **Kaposi's sarcoma**.

There is no cure for AIDS; the most effective 'remedy' is avoidance of infection. In recent years a number of drugs have been discovered that may be effective in allowing HIV infected people to live longer lives. The major problems associated with the current drugs are:

- Significant toxicity through prolonged usage or high doses, e.g. **azidothymidine** (**AZT**; a nucleoside analogue that inhibits tran-scription of viral RNA into DNA by targeting the reverse transcriptase enzyme) can also inhibit normal leukocyte proliferation.
- The development of resistant variants of the HIV virus because of its very high mutation rate, e.g. individual **protease inhibitors** may prove effective for a time by preventing final assembly of new viral particles, however resistance develops rapidly. A solution which shows promise is to use combinations, or cock-tails, of several different forms of these two types of drugs.

Some degree of immune suppression is a common finding in the aftermath of a number of viral infections, e.g. chicken pox or measles. The precise mechanisms underlying these phenomena are unknown.

Table 9.2   *Clinical and laboratory indices leading to a diagnosis of AIDS*

Laboratory index	Level
CD4$^+$ T cell number	200 or less per mm^3 of blood
CD4$^+$: CD8$^+$	0.5 or less
HIV RNA	Sharply increased
β$_2$-microglobulin	Increased (paediatric AIDS)
Neopterin (a macrophage product)	Increased

When AIDS is diagnosed patients usually have one or more of the following:

Infections with:
  Cryptosporidium
  Cryptococcus
  Herpes Simplex Virus (HSV)
  Cytomegalovirus (CMV)
  Leptospora
  Histoplasma
  Mycobacterium avium
  Mycobacterium tuberculosis
  Pneumocystis carinii
  Toxoplasma

Malignancy:
  Kaposi's syndrome
  Lymphoma (Burkitt's or other type)

Other diseases:
  Encephalopathy
  Wasting syndrome

Suggested further reading

Day, M. (1998) Guerrilla warfare. *New Scientist* 160, 32–37.

Edwards-Jones, V. and Shawcross, S.G. (1997) Toxic shock syndrome in the burned patient. *British Journal of Biomedical Science* 54, 110–117.

Elgert, K.D., Alleva, D.G. and Mullins, D.W. (1998) Tumor-induced immune dysfunction: the macrophage connection. *Journal of Leukocyte Biology* 64, 275–290.

Feinberg, M.B. (1996) Changing the natural history of HIV disease. *Lancet* 348, 239–246.

Fischer, A., Cavazzana-Calvo, M., DeSaint Basile, G., DeVollartay, J.P., Disanto, J.P., Hirroz, C., Rieux-Laucat, F. and LeDiest, F. (1997) Naturally occurring primary deficiencies of the immune system. *Annual Review of Immunology* 15, 93–124.

George, A.J.T. and Ritter, M.A. (1996) Thymic involution with ageing: obsolescence or good housekeeping? *Immunology Today* 17, 267–271.

Horuk, R. (1999) Chemokine receptors and HIV-1: the fusion of two major research fields. *Immunology Today* 20, 89–94.

Knight, S.C. and Patterson, S. (1997) Bone marrow-derived dendritic cells, infection with human immunodeficiency virus, and immunopathology. *Annual Review of Immunology* 15, 593–616.

Mattsson, P.T., Vihinen, M. and Smith, C.I.E. (1996) X-linked agammaglobulinaemia (XLA): a genetic tyrosine kinase (Btk) disease. *Bioessays* 18, 825–834.

Nobel, G.J. (1999) A transformed view of cyclosporine. *Nature* 397, 471–472.

Pawelec, G., Solana, R., Remarque, E. and Mariani, E. (1998) Impact of ageing on innate immunity. *Journal of Leukocyte Biology* 64, 703–712.

Resta, R. and Thompson, L.F. (1997) SCID: the role of adenosine deaminase deficiency. *Immunology Today* 18, 371–374.

Rodewald, H-R. (1998) The thymus in the age of retirement. *Nature* 396, 630–631.

Spickett, G.P., Farrant, J., North, M.E., Zhang, J-G., Morgan, L. and Webster, A.D.B. (1997) Common variable immunodeficiency; how many diseases? *Immunology Today* 18, 325–328.

Thomas, M. and Brady, L. (1997) HIV integrase: a target for AIDS therapies. *Trends in Biotechnology* 15, 167–172.

Self-assessment questions

1. A 43-year old female has a 5-year history of recurrent bacterial infections. Laboratory tests suggest that her IgG and IgA levels are decreased while IgM is normal. Which B cell deficiency condition is likely to be present? Explain your answer.

2. In which Ig deficiency disease is IgM particularly elevated?

3. In children, which Ig isotype takes the longest time to achieve adult levels?

4. In which condition is thymic deficiency found together with parathyroid abnormalities?

5. Why is it vital to remove passenger lymphocytes from bone marrow grafts to SCID children?

6. What enzyme is defective in chronic granulomatous disease patients and what cellular function is impaired as a consequence?

7. List three factors that may predispose to immunosenescence.

8. Which of the following ratios of $CD4^+$ to $CD8^+$ T cells would you expect to find in a patient with AIDS?

   a. 1.5
   b. 2.0
   c. 5.0
   d. 0.5

9. List two possible ways in which anti-HIV antibodies may alter the course of the infection.

10. Once the initial phase of the illness has passed, HIV-infected people exhibit low numbers of infected T cells in the circulation. However we now know that a significant load of viruses may still be present in the body. Where are these viruses?

Key Concepts and Facts

Immune Deficiency
- Deficiencies may be primary or secondary; congenital (inborn) or acquired.

- Primary deficiencies are those in which the defect is within the immune system itself. Defects in any component of the immune system may lead to deficiency.

- Secondary immune deficiencies occur as a result of a disease process or damage to some other body system which then impacts upon the mechanisms or products of the immune system.

Deficiencies of B Cells
- Many B cell deficiencies are known and may be detected as decreased levels of all, or some, immunoglobulin isotypes.

- B cell deficiencies lead to recurrent infections usually with bacteria.

- Many B cell deficiencies may be treated with repeated injections with immunoglobulins.

Deficiencies of T Cells
- Immune deficiencies associated with T cells are rare, probably due to the essential role of T cells, hence deficient patients would succumb rapidly to infection.

- Common infections in T cell deficient patients are viral or fungal.

Combined B cell and T cell Deficiencies
- These have the most serious consequence for the patient.

- Babies born with SCID usually die from massive infections by the age of 2 years although, now, bone marrow transplants are proving successful.

Secondary Immune Deficiencies
- Causes include: ageing, malignancy, nutritional deficiencies, exposure to radiation, burns, immunosuppressive therapies (and other chemotherapies) and viral infections, e.g. HIV/AIDS.

- All CD4$^+$ cells are targets for the HIV virus, however only CD4$^+$ T cells are killed.

- Cytotoxic T cells provide effective defence against HIV for many years following infection. However the persistence of viral proliferation and a high mutation rate eventually allow the HIV to gain the upper hand and proceed to destroy all CD4$^+$ T cells, leaving the patient susceptible to a wide range of infectious agents.

Chapter 10
Immunology: applications

Learning objectives

After studying this chapter you should confidently be able to:

Discuss the application of immunology to modern diagnostic techniques.

Describe the use of immunological molecules as technological tools.

Discuss the current use and future potential of immunological reagents in the treatment of human diseases.

Assays based upon the unique features of immune system cells and molecules are now very important in laboratories devoted to the diagnosis of human or animal diseases. The diseases investigated do not necessarily originate in immune systems, although they may. Biological assays that exploit immune cells or antibodies (in practice it is most frequently antibodies) are known as **immunoassays**.

For all antibody-based diagnostic systems the principal constraint is the availability of an appropriate antibody reagent. For many years tests were performed using antibodies raised by the injection of soluble antigen into an animal. The antibodies were then harvested by collecting the blood plasma from the animal. These antibodies were known as **polyclonal antibodies** because the population of antibodies recovered would include the products of many different reacting B cell clones (Figure 10.1). The antibodies against the injected antigen would be likely to be present in relatively high concentration, however many other antibodies of different specificity would also be present. It was always possible for some of these other antibodies to react with antigens in the relevant test and so produce misleading results. Further, the quality control mechanisms necessary to ensure some level of consistency between different batches of antibody preparations were difficult to improve upon. To enhance the quality and usefulness of the immunological reagents available for diagnostic tests it would be necessary to produce homogeneous antibodies all known to be specific for a single antigenic determinant and present in high concentration in reproducible batches. The great similarity in protein structure

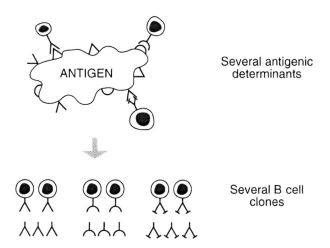

Figure 10.1 *This is a polyclonal antibody preparation because the population of antibodies includes the products of many different B cell clones*

Several antigenic determinants

Several B cell clones

between one antibody and another meant that a solution could not be found in biochemical purification.

The technical advance in cell fusion made by Kohler and Milstein in 1975 led to the production of permanent cell lines producing antibody specific for a predetermined antigen. These antibodies were known as **monoclonal antibodies (MABs)**.

The basis of the production process for MABs is that single antibody-secreting B cells are fused with immortal cell lines. These immortal cells are usually myelomas, i.e. transformed B cells. It is important for the myeloma cells to have lost the ability to secrete antibody. The fusion product is both immortal and produces antibody of the desired specificity. These hybrids can be cultured to produce a clone of identical antibody-secreting cells. Such a clone is known as a **hybridoma**. Through several well-defined stages it is possible to isolate large quantities of highly pure, specific antibodies produced by the hybridomas (Figure 10.2), i.e. the MAB.

The traditional starting-point of the MAB production procedure is still the injection of antigen into an animal. However advances in molecular biology have led to antibody engineering techniques in which isolated antibody genes can be manipulated. With the ready availability of MABs a revolution in diagnostic testing has taken place.

Immunoassays exploit the specificity of binding between antibodies and antigens. In the simplest possible terms, an immunoassay can use a known antibody to detect the presence of an antigen whether it is a component of a tissue, an isolated cell or is a soluble molecule. Recognizing that all antibodies are protein (or glycoprotein) in nature, it is then possible to use a known antibody to detect the presence of an antigen or another antibody. These measurements that give essentially 'Yes' or 'No' answers ('Yes' the target molecule is present or 'No' the target molecule is not present) are know as **qualitative** tests. By very careful control of the test

Kohler and Milstein were immunologists working on a fundamental question. They wanted to be able to prove whether single B cells produced antibody of only a single specificity. In order to do this they had to find a way to produce large quantities of antibody that would be the product of only a single B cell. Once they had achieved this goal, they realized that their work might have further application to techniques and procedures that required large quantities of specific antibody. Their findings were published in the journal Nature and led to the award of a Nobel prize.

Figure 10.2 *A scheme for the production of monoclonal antibodies using 'conventional' technology*

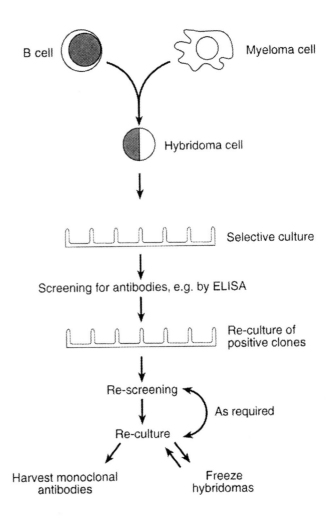

B cell

Myeloma cell

Hybridoma cell

Selective culture

Screening for antibodies, e.g. by ELISA

Re-culture of positive clones

Re-screening

As required

Re-culture

Harvest monoclonal antibodies

Freeze hybridomas

A test platform is most easily considered as the type of basic technology that underpins the test and allows data to be generated. The same term is often used in relation to computers: PC and Macintosh are the most common computer platforms. Both can be used to perform essentially similar tasks, however the two operating systems are different.

The first study using immunohistochemistry was reported in 1942. It involved the use of a fluorescent dye to label pneumococcal antigens in infected tissues.

conditions, it is possible to use immunoassays to answer questions about how much of a target antigen or antibody is present. These are known as **quantitative** tests.

Antibody-based immunoassays have many advantages over conventional biochemical tests. Some of these advantages are:

- increased specificity;
- increased sensitivity;
- increased flexibility of test platform.

The most common test platforms are: immunohistochemistry, immunocytochemistry, radioimmunoassay (RIA) and enzyme-linked immunosorbent assay (ELISA).

The use of specific antibodies to probe for the presence of an antigen in a section of tissue is **immunohistochemistry** while **immunocytochemistry** probes for antigen in isolated cell populations. The principle underlying both sets of techniques is identical

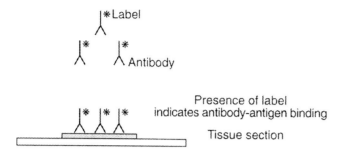

Figure 10.3 *The label bound to the antibody marks each site of antibody-antigen binding*

and, in practice, the two terms are used interchangeably. In general they combine histological, immunological and biochemical techniques. They build upon, and can be used in a complementary manner to, conventional tincture-based (colorimetric) stains. These stains bind chemically to particular components of cells or tissues generally showing a consistent pattern of staining wherever a particular type of biochemical molecule occurs, e.g. a stain for protein will produce a similar pattern whatever the precise nature of the protein. The interpretation of conventional histological staining patterns is a highly skilled task requiring a great deal of experience combined with intuition and deduction. When using immunological reagents however, particular characteristics of different protein molecules can be highlighted so that they appear distinct, i.e. different proteins are regarded as different antigens.

The presence of any antigen can be determined once you have an antibody reagent specific for that antigen. A potential technical challenge is posed by the fact that antigen–antibody binding is colourless. Specialized techniques must be used to indicate that binding has taken place. This visualization is achieved by adding a marker, or label to the reagent antibody. With the label attached to the antibody, everywhere label is detected correlates with a site where an antibody has bound to an antigen (Figure 10.3). The antibody labels that have been used to-date are:

- radioisotopes;
- fluorochromes, i.e. molecules that fluoresce at a particular wavelength (i.e. colour) when they are exposed to UV light;
- enzymes.

Of these, the use of radioisotopes is now rare due to the necessary health and safety precautions together with the need for specialized handling facilities. Fluorochromes also are used less frequently than previously for the staining of tissue sections or cell preparations. This is largely because of the transience of the results – the colour produced on exposure to UV gradually bleaches over time. The bleaching effect requires that much of the work is carried out under conditions where the sample under examination can be kept in the dark. In addition the analysis of sections that have been stained

Although one of the big advantages of enzyme-linked immunohistochemistry is that the results can be visualized under light microscopy, there is also the option of using an electron-dense label for electron microscopy. One material that is used in this way is colloidal gold. Under electron microscopy (EM) structures that have been stained with colloidal gold may be identified by the presence of distinct dark 'dots' at the sites of antibody binding. The gold particles cannot be seen under light microscopy, however their enhancement by silver does allow them to be observed. This particular technique requires very special attention to eliminating any contaminating metals that might be in the reagent solutions.

with a fluorochrome requires the use of a specialized UV microscope. The use of fluorochromes is now extensive however in the technique of flow cytometry as carried out using a fluorescence activated cell sorter (FACS). The most widely used fluorochromes are FITC (**fluorescein** isothiocyanate) which gives a green fluorescence and **rhodamine** isothiocyanate (red fluorescence).

Enzyme-linked systems are now the most commonplace in immunohistochemistry. The principle of the technique is that an enzyme is conjugated (bound chemically) to an antibody. Each site where an antibody binds will also carry a molecule of enzyme. The enzymes chosen are those that react with a substrate to produce a coloured product. The location of the coloured product is the site where antigen–antibody binding has taken place and the patterns observed are usually clear and distinct. By combining this approach with image analysis systems, i.e. computerized systems for analysis of microscopical images, the results can be made semi-quantitative, the amount of antigen present correlating with the extent and/or density of the antibody staining. Enzymes that have been used in immunohistochemistry include **horseradish peroxidase** (brown staining) and **alkaline phosphatase** (red staining).

The major advantages of enzyme-linked immunostaining methods are that:

- the end result is generally long-lasting;
- the results can be viewed under simple light microscope;
- no particular health and safety precautions are necessary.

The most important consideration when preparing antibody-labelled conjugates is that the conjugation should not affect the antibody's binding activity. Chemical methods such as cyanogen bromide treatment may be used, however the biologically based **avidin–biotin** system is now popular. Avidin and biotin are a pair of molecules that bind together with exceptionally high affinity so their interaction is stable at extremes of temperature, pH, etc. Biotin is a water-soluble vitamin and avidin is a protein component of egg white. It is also found in microorganisms so in fact this **streptavidin** is commonly used. When an antibody is conjugated to avidin, the label that is bound to biotin will attach strongly to the avidin. Avidin is a tetramer of four identical binding sites for biotin therefore amplification through the binding of multiple biotinylated (biotin-conjugated) ligands is possible. The avidin–biotin complex (ABC) method uses a biotinylated enzyme label that is pre-incubated with avidin. This forms large complexes that can then be incubated with a biotinylated antibody (Figure 10.4).

Good conjugation systems have yielded a method by which the 'signal' derived from the binding of an antibody with an antigen can be amplified many-fold. Figure 10.5 shows that many molecules of label can be attached to an antibody. This technique is known as **direct immunohistochemistry**. In Figure 10.6 amplification can be

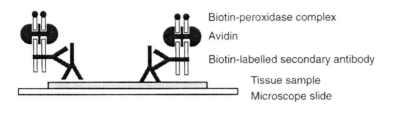

Biotin-peroxidase complex
Avidin
Biotin-labelled secondary antibody
Tissue sample
Microscope slide

Figure 10.4 *The avidin–biotin complex (ABC) method*

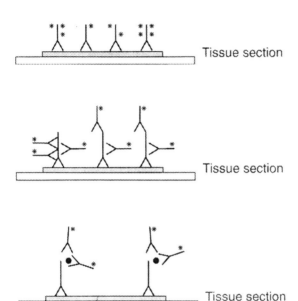

Tissue section

Figure 10.5 *Direct immunocytochemistry: amplification of the signal from antibody–antigen binding by attachment of multiple molecules of label to an antibody*

Tissue section

Figure 10.6 *Indirect immunocytochemistry: further amplification of an antigen–antibody binding signal is achieved using a secondary antibody*

Tissue section

Figure 10.7 *Indirect immunocytochemistry: secondary antibodies are directed against an enzyme label in systems such as PAP, APAAP or GAG*

seen to involve the use of a secondary antibody. Several molecules of the secondary antibody will bind to the primary antibody, i.e. the antibody specific for the antigen of interest. Such systems involving secondary antibodies are now used extensively and are termed **indirect immunohistochemistry**. More layers of antibody can be used to provide further amplification however this is limited by the risk of inducing non-specific effects as the total amount of protein loaded onto the section is increased.

Additional refinements of enzyme-linked systems have involved the use of secondary antibodies directed against the enzyme label. Examples of such a system are **PAP** (peroxidase–anti peroxidase), **APAAP** (alkaline phosphatase–anti-alkaline phosphatase) and **GAG** (glucose oxidase–anti-glucose oxidase) (Figure 10.7). The principal advantage of these systems is the ability to load the amount of label on the third layer. A secondary antibody acts as a linker between the primary and tertiary layers. The overall complex is highly stable and allows for a very high label-to-primary antibody ratio. Where the amount of primary antibody used can be kept low, the chances of non-specific effects can be reduced. The main disadvantage of the method, apart from the additional steps that must be performed, is

The avidin–biotin complex (ABC) method has been reported to be some 40 times more sensitive than the PAP method and is also considerably faster to complete. The need to block endogenous avidin and the reduced penetration of the large complexes into tissues are the principal disadvantages.

that it may be difficult for the large complex to penetrate into the tissues.

Whichever immunohistochemical visualization system (label) is used there are some basic technical principles that must be observed if the technique is to be effective:

- the **morphology** of the tissues and cells must be retained;
- the **antigenicity** must be preserved and unchanged;
- the antigenic sites must be accessible.

Correct **fixation** of the tissue or cell sample is essential because inappropriate fixation can lead to the destruction of antigenic sites or make the tissue impenetrable to the reagent antibody. Fixation is necessary because it arrests tissue activities such as diffusion of soluble components or enzymatic activity, it prevents tissue decomposition and it gives the tissue some protection against the various stages in the immunostaining procedure. The ideal fixative differs from tissue to tissue and from antigen to antigen. The sectioning of the tissue can be done in several different ways, most frequently paraffin sections or cryostat (frozen) sections. Once again care must be taken in the selection of the method as some reagent antibodies work optimally on particular types of section.

Despite the careful selection of processing techniques it is sometimes still necessary to 'unmask' antigens within a tissue section. This can also help to remove unwanted background staining. While the molecular basis of unmasking is not fully understood, procedures that are used to bring it about include limited proteolytic digestion with enzymes such as chymotrypsin or trypsin and the application of microwaves.

A further consideration when using enzyme-labelling methods is the possible presence of **endogenous enzyme** within the tissue or cell sample. For example, if horseradish peroxidase is being used as the label the substrate that is added to detect antibody binding can also be converted to product by the peroxidase activity of tissue haemoproteins and catalases. If these react with the substrate they produce a high level of non-specific background staining that is difficult to distinguish from the specific staining. Fortunately it is possible to destroy the endogenous activity during the processing. Endogenous peroxidase can be destroyed by 3% hydrogen peroxide, however the procedure used must be such that there is no risk of the endogenous inhibitor affecting the label that is attached to the antibody. For some tissues that are especially rich in peroxidase activity an alternative enzyme label should be used. If avidin–biotin is being used as a conjugation system care must be taken with tissues that may be rich in biotin, e.g. liver, mammary gland, adipose tissue or kidney.

For all techniques, non-specific binding sites must be blocked. This involves the application of a solution that will adhere to protein-binding sites on the section. Normal serum is frequently

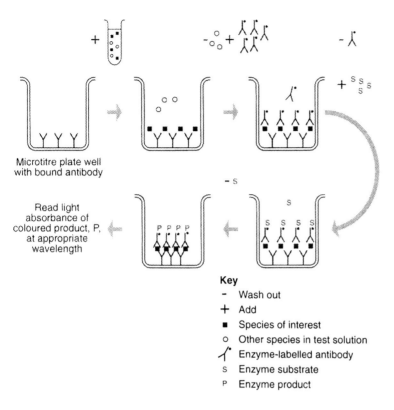

Figure 10.8 *ELISA: a frequently-used immunoassay technique*

Microtitre plate well
with bound antibody

Read light
absorbance of
coloured product, P,
at appropriate
wavelength

Key

-   Wash out
+   Add
■   Species of interest
○   Other species in test solution
⅄   Enzyme-labelled antibody
s   Enzyme substrate
P   Enzyme product

used as the **blocking agent** but care must be taken to ensure that the species of origin of the serum will not induce further unwanted interactions with the primary or secondary antibody. A useful strategy often is to use normal serum from the same species as the primary antibody.

Both **radioimmunoassay (RIA)** and **enzyme-linked immunosorbent assay (ELISA)** also exploit the specific interactions of antibodies with antigens. They differ from immunohistochemical techniques in that they are used to detect and quantify soluble molecules. Labelled antibodies are used to capture the antigen of interest that can then be measured either in a supernatant or bound to a solid support, most usually the wells of a microtitre plate. Here also the use of radioisotopes has declined so that ELISA is now by far the more frequently used version of the technique (Figure 10.8). As when using labelled antibody reagents in immunohistochemistry, the ELISA reagents can be used in many different conformations so as to optimize the measurement of the antigen of interest. With the use of standardized, commercial ELISA microtitre plates many of the problems encountered when using tissue sections are eliminated, e.g. the only blocking that is usually necessary is of positively charged sites on the plastic surface of microtitre wells. This is readily blocked by the addition of protein solutions. Once again, however, the most stringent preparatory tests must be

Figure 10.9 *Detection of fluorescently-labelled cells by FACS*

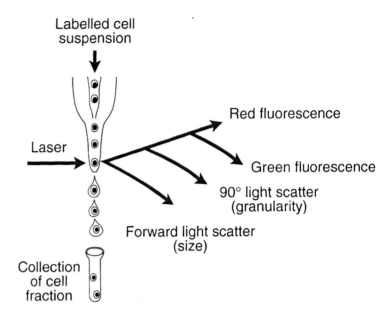

undertaken in order to optimize every stage in the procedure. Microtitre plate ELISA uses very small quantities both of reagents and of samples and many of the steps in the assay can be automated through the use of automatic place washers, reagent dispensers and plate readers. Very high throughput of samples for a wide range of different tests has been made possible through the widespread availability and use of ELISA.

The advent of **fluorescence activated cell sorting (FACS)** has allowed the high throughput of samples that is seen with ELISA to be extended to the analysis of cell populations. Conventionally when fluorochrome-labelled antibodies bind to cells, their presence is detected visually with UV microscopy. This is time-consuming and subject to operator-dependent error. The FACS machine allows fluorescently labelled cell populations to be enumerated and, if desired, to be separated into individual populations. The FACS machine uses a laser to detect cells that fluoresce at particular wavelengths (Figure 10.9). The proportion of cells in a population showing a particular pattern of fluorescence can be enumerated and the data displayed (Figure 10.10). Cell populations to be analysed can be reacted with two or three different antibodies in a single test allowing the simultaneous display of data on two or three different cell types. These are known as two-colour or three-colour fluorescence, respectively. Very careful optimization of the test conditions is necessary for multiple investigations and the manipulation of the data on three-colour fluorescence studies can be complex.

Immunotechnology is a growing and important industry worldwide. The production of immunological reagents whether for use *in vitro* or *in vivo* is a core component of the industry.

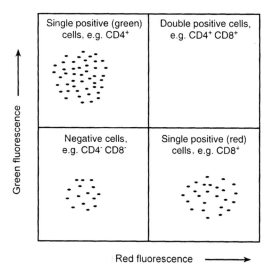

Figure 10.10 *Diagrammatic representation of information on cells that can be generated by FACS*

Immunotherapy, the manipulation of the immune response *in vivo*, is made possible by the availability of high quality immunological reagents.

When MABs were first developed, great interest was stimulated in their potential for *in vivo* use. The concept was that these antibodies could be used to target drug treatments within the body and so avoid the possibility of side-effects. The drug of choice could be conjugated to the antibody which would then function as a 'magic bullet' to direct the attached drug to its proposed site of action. The treatment of cancer, where side-effects typically are a major limiting factor for the use of the treatment, might have been revolutionized by such techniques. To-date, however, monoclonal antibody therapy has not achieved its anticipated potential. There are a number of reasons for this including:

- The conjugation process could alter the antibody specificity or reduce the effectiveness of the drug.

- The conjugation process would have to be very effective to ensure the drug would not be released at microenvironments within the body with extremes, e.g. of pH.

- No definite tumour-specific antigens are known against which a specific MAB could be raised. Further, many tumour cells tend to shed their surface antigens more frequently than normal cells. When the antigens reappear they may be different to the original.

- Even if a MAB–drug conjugate reached the tumour site, its incorporation into the target tumour cell could not be guaranteed.

- Repeated administration of the antibody–drug conjugate would be required to induce an effective response. As the monoclonal

Figure 10.11 *Humanization of murine monoclonal antibodies to reduce the risk of HAMA response*

 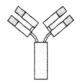

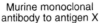

| Murine monoclonal antibody to antigen X | Human monoclonal antibody to antigen X | Humanized monoclonal antibody to antigen X |

antibodies are generally raised in mice, they are murine proteins and so become targets of the human immune response. This human anti-mouse antibody response (HAMA) can destroy the antibody–drug conjugate and may lead to disorders in the patient associated with large amounts of immune complexes in the circulation.

In an attempt to overcome the HAMA response murine antibodies have been humanized (Figure 10.11) by transplanting the antigen-binding sites of murine MABs onto a framework provided by human antibodies. Thus there is only a very small murine target to be identified by the patient's immune system and the HAMA response is reduced. Humanized antibodies are currently undergoing clinical trials.

Monoclonal antibodies are also used as aids in the visualization of tumours within the body, especially either prior to or following surgery for cancer. Antibodies raised against a tumour type can be labelled with a stable isotope, e.g. Indium 111, and injected into the patient. A large fraction of the labelled antibody localizes to the site of a tumour and can be visualized using an appropriate body scanner. This will allow clinicians to:

- visualize the location of a tumour relative to vital organs or tissues;
- decide whether or not initial surgery has effectively removed the tumour tissue;
- see whether secondary tumours may be present distant from the primary site.

Other immunological reagents apart from MABs may also be used in attempts to manipulate *in vivo* immune responses. Most human tumours do not elicit a detectable host immune response so it is valuable to attempt to manipulate the immune system in such a way as to promote anti-tumour responses.

Adoptive immunotherapy is a form of therapy in which immune cells are transferred to patients with cancer. The immune cells are directed specifically towards the patient's tumour. The initial phases of the treatment involve the collection of leukocytes from the patient (leukopheresis) and the acseptic *in vitro* culture of the leukocytes in the presence of high concentrations of IL-2. The

When a patient has received a radiolabelled antibody the clinician can track how the localization of the radiolabel within the body changes over time. Gradually the majority of the label will be seen to associate with the liver. This does not always mean that the patient has a tumour in the liver but that the body's normal clearance mechanism for proteins, or detoxification, is underway.

IL-2 treatment causes the leukocytes to proliferate through several cycles of replication and to differentiate into **lymphokine-activated killer (LAK) cells**. As well as possessing cytotoxic activity, the cells also express the IL-2 receptor therefore will continue to expand in the presence of IL-2. Some 10^{10} or 10^{11} leukocytes are needed for a single patient treatment. These 'expanded' cell populations are then re-infused into the patient from whom they were originally collected together with the lowest possible maintenance dose of IL-2. Types of tumours that have been treated using adoptive immunotherapy include melanoma and renal carcinoma. Perhaps the most effective use of this procedure is in patients whose tumour burden has been decreased by surgery or in whom the disease is in the early stage of relapse. A number of complete or partial recoveries have been documented for tumours that had proved resistant to the conventional treatments of chemotherapy and radiotherapy, however LAK cell treatment is still rather less effective than was originally hoped.

There are many potential hazards in IL-2/LAK therapy. Some areas in which particular care is required include:

- Avoiding the risk of contamination of the leukocytes during collection, culture or re-infusion.

- The high toxicity of IL-2. Early treatments with IL-2 involved direct infusion of the cytokine into the patient, however the toxicity was overwhelming due to the high doses required. The procedure has to be carried out in an intensive care unit. The symptoms of IL-2 toxicity include: fever, diarrhoea, thrombocytopenia, pulmonary oedema, confusion (sleepiness, disorientation, depression), insomnia and coma.

- The potential for the re-infused LAK cells to migrate to other body sites apart from the tumour, e.g. lung, liver and spleen, and causing damage to these otherwise healthy tissues.

Refinements of LAK/IL-2 treatment include the use of **tumour-infiltrating lymphocytes (TIL)** instead of circulating leukocytes. While this modification may increase the likelihood of the re-infused cells migrating to the tumour site, and allow the cells to respond specifically to tumour cells to which they have previously been exposed, a new difficulty is created. This is the need to extract the viable TIL from the patient's excised tumour tissue. Combinations of physical and enzymatic disruption of the tumour are used. The development of treatment protocols whereby IL-2 could be used to induce LAK *in vivo* would obviate this very troublesome stage. A further refinement is the introduction of the gene for a cytokine directly into tumour cells.

Cytokines, e.g. TNF-α, clearly have the potential to kill tumour cells. However the initial promise of such treatments has never been achieved, principally because of the accompanying inherent toxicity of the cytokine towards normal host cells. The condition known as **cachexia** is the severe metabolic disturbances and muscle wasting that is characteristic of advanced cancer. It is TNF-α that also induces this life-threatening condition. It has been an unfulfilled goal of immunologists to manipulate the TNF protein in such as way as to retain its anti-tumour activity while deleting its cachectic function. Numerous studies over the years have suggested that the use of single cytokines for therapy is unlikely to be beneficial. Combinations of a number of cytokines that more closely resemble the *in vivo* situation may prove more effective, however the precise constituents of such a cytokine cocktail or the optimal concentrations of each cytokine are as yet unknown.

The susceptibility of tumours to the induced immune responses may also be increased. Most tumour cells typically express very low numbers of MHC molecules hence are less likely to be targets of T cells. Inducing the increased expression of MHC Class I molecules on the tumour cells may render them more immunogenic.

Some very definite success with the use of cytokines has been achieved with specific cancer types. Interferon alpha-2 (IFN-α_2) has been used to treat chronic myelogenous leukaemia and other myeloproliferative disorders. Used in combination with retinoids, IFN-α_2 has induced regression in advanced squamous carcinomas of the skin and cervix. It also has been useful in the treatment of melanomas, hypernephromas, and haemangiomas. There are at least 15 different molecular species of IFN-α. A number of these are available as recombinant products, however the process of clinical testing of all available variants of the cytokine against neoplastic diseases has a very long way to go.

The use of **gene therapy** to manipulate immune responses *in vivo* is now being attempted. For example, cytokine gene therapy may become a useful complement to conventional treatments (surgery, chemotherapy, radiotherapy) and may permit effective vaccination against cancer under safe clinical conditions. The transfer of cytokine genes is based on the use of targeted **gene delivery vectors** (e.g. replication-deficient retroviruses, HSV vectors or adenovirus vectors). These vectors introduce and stably express cloned cytokine genes (or the corresponding cytokine receptor genes) into the genomes of tumour cell lines, immune cells or haematopoietic stem cells. This procedure generates cells that overexpress the transferred gene in a controlled manner. The goal is to guarantee the prolonged release of elevated quantities of cytokines in the tumour microenvironment, in order to achieve local responses without systemic toxicities. Where a cytokine receptor gene is transferred, it is the tumour cell's response to cytokines that is upregulated. At present the patients who are eligible for experimental treatments such as cytokine gene transfer therapy are those with cancer that has failed all standard treatment and for which no other effective treatment options are available.

Suggested further reading

Borrebaeck, C.A.K. (1995) Antibody Engineering. Oxford: Oxford University Press.

Franks, L.M. and Teich, N.M. (1997) Introduction to the Cellular and Molecular Biology of Cancer. Oxford: Oxford University Press.

Hall, S.S. (1997) A Commotion in the Blood. New York: Henry Holt.

Johnston, A. and Turner, M. (1997) Immunochemistry: A Practical Approach. Oxford: Oxford University Press.

Kohler, G. and Milstein, C. (1975) *Nature* **256**, 495–498.

Leong, S.S.-Y., Cooper, K., Joel, F. and Leong, W.-M. (1998) Manual of Diagnostic Antibodies for Immunohistology. Oxford: Oxford University Press.

Old, L.J. (1996) Immunotherapy for Cancer. *Scientific American*, **275**, 136–143.

Rosenberg, S.A. (1992) The Transformed Cell. London: Phoenix Paperbacks.

Self-assessment questions

1. Distinguish between polyclonal and monoclonal antibodies.
2. List three advantages of immunoassays over conventional biochemical tests.
3. Explain the principle of the ABC method of immunohistochemistry.
4. What is the main advantage of indirect immunohistochemistry over direct methods?
5. Why may it be necessary to block endogenous peroxidase activity within a tissue undergoing immunohistochemical investigation?
6. What is a 'sandwich' ELISA?
7. List the possible side-effects of high dose IL-2 treatment.
8. What causes a HAMA response?
9. What are LAK cells?
10. The *in vivo* use of which cytokine is limited because it induces the pathological muscle-wasting known as cachexia?

Key Concepts and Facts

Monoclonal Antibodies
- Fusion of an antibody-producing B cell and a myeloma cell produces an immortal antibody-producing cell. A clone of these cells is known as a hybridoma.

- Monoclonal antibodies are highly purified preparations of antibody of a single specificity.

- Monoclonal antibodies can be produced in large quantities to produce high quality diagnostic reagents.

Immunohistochemistry
- Has many advantages over traditional colorimetric histological techniques.

- Produces results that are clear and readily interpreted.

Enzyme-linked Immunosorbent Assay (ELISA)
- Is the basis for tests that are highly specific, reliable and economical.

- Automation of the ELISA procedure allows for very high throughput of assays.

Manipulation of the Immune System In Vivo
- Monoclonal antibodies appear to hold great promise for targeting of treatments *in vivo*, however that promise has proven difficult to realize.

- Adoptive immunotherapy for cancer involves the manipulation of immune cells outside of the body and their re-infusion into the patient. These cells should then be able to generate more effective anti-tumour responses.

- Gene therapy may be used to introduce cytokine genes directly into tumour cells. The genes are then expressed to ensure prolonged local release of the cytokine.

Answers to self-assessment questions

Chapter 1

1.

Acute inflammation	Chronic inflammation
Rapid	Long-lasting
Beneficial	Disease process that damages the host

2.

Natural immune responses	Acquired immune responses
Inborn	Develop throughout life as they are permanently changed on every encounter with non-self
Unchanging	Memory
Non-specific	Specific

3. Immune response.
4. Phagocytosis.
5. Vascular endothelial cells.
6. Recurrent infections. The severity of the infections is determined by the nature and extent of the immune deficiency.
7. Autoimmune diseases involve immune responses that are directed against components of the host.
8. HIV: human immunodeficiency virus;
   AIDS: acquired immune deficiency syndrome.
9. One or more of: multiple infections, cancer, dementia.
10. Immunization.

Chapter 2

1. Active bone marrow is not present in the long (limb) bones of the adult and the adult thymus has shrunken to microscopic size.

2. The lymphatic vessels collect fluid that enters the tissue from the arterial system and return it to the cardiovascular system at the subclavian vein; white blood cells circulate in the blood and in the lymph; the locations of lymphatic vessels parallel those of the veins.

3. The polymorphonuclear leukocytes (PMNs) comprise neutrophils, basophils and eosinophils. Their nucleus is multi-lobed and they contain cytoplasmic granules. Mononuclear phagocytes are circulating monocytes and macrophages and macrophage-like cells within the tissues. Their nucleus is approximately spherical and cytoplasmic granules are not apparent under light microscopy.

4. Neutrophils are the most abundant leukocyte type within the circulating blood. The normal count is between 3000 and 6000 cells per mL of blood, i.e. 60% of all circulating leukocytes.

5. Lymphoid tissues are found adjacent to the interfaces where self and non-self are most likely to make contact. These include the mucosal surfaces, e.g. linings of the digestive, respiratory and genito-urinary tracts; and the spleen and lymph nodes where non-self may be filtered from lymph and blood, respectively.

6. B lymphocytes, or B cells, were named after the organ called the Bursa of Fabricius that is found in birds and is the site of B cell maturation. In mammals B cell maturation occurs in the bone marrow. T lymphocytes, or T cells, complete their maturation within the thymus (T = thymus).

7. The liver is the principal site of APP synthesis. The Major APP are those whose concentration increases greatly (about 1000-fold) during the acute phase of immune responses. Two Major APPs are C-reactive protein (CRP) and serum amyloid A (SAA).

8. Cytokines interact with specific receptors on the surface of target cells. When the receptor is occupied by the appropriate cytokine the cell's response is initiated.

9. Cytokines must reach a particular concentration (usually in the nanomolar or picomolar range) before they have an effect although excessively high concentrations may be very dangerous; cytokine antagonists have also been identified and they can inhibit the effects of cytokines.

10. Cells that are cultured in laboratories are maintained in fluid known as cell culture medium. Following a period of culture this medium was separated from the cells. The medium was then added to a separate group of cells (target cells) and these cells were seen to respond in particular ways. The responses could not be induced using fresh culture medium in which cells had not previously been grown. Biochemical methods of protein separation were used to purify the molecules responsible for the effects on the target cells. These molecules were what we now call cytokines.

Chapter 3

1. Swelling, redness, pain and heat.
2. FMLP is a sequence of the amino acids formylmethionine, leucine and phenylalanine that is produced when bacterial protein synthesis occurs. In host tissues FMLP acts as an inflammatory mediator.
3. Aspirin inhibits the enzyme cyclo-oxygenase thereby preventing the synthesis of a range of eicosanoids. It is one of the group of non-steroidal anti-inflammatory drugs (NSAIDs).
4. Endothelial cells change shape causing gaps between adjacent cells, they become 'sticky' by the expression of cell surface adhesion molecules and they express cytokines that increase the rate and extent of inflammatory responses.
5. Chemotaxis is directional cell movement along a chemical gradient. It is the process by which infiltrating leukocytes move through the tissues to the site where the foreign body is present.
6. Opsonization is the enhancement of phagocytosis that occurs when opsonins, e.g. complement factors, are attached to the surface of target cells.
7. The enzyme NADPH oxidase catalyses the respiratory burst of phagocytes. Neutrophils also contain the enzyme myeloperoxidase that catalyses the interaction of ROS with halogens to produce new, highly-reactive chemicals such as hypochloric acid (HOCl).
8. The liver is the principal target organ of pro-inflammatory cytokines.
9. Complement factor C3 is vital because it is a key component of all pathways of complement activation. It is also the most abundant of the complement proteins. A person born with severe C3 deficiency would suffer recurrent infections, predominantly bacterial. Complete absence of C3 usually is not compatible with life.
10. The sequence of wound healing stages is: activation of the blood clotting cascade; colonization of the fibrin clot by inflammatory cells; platelet degranulation; inactivation of clotting factors; dissolution of the thrombus; further migration of inflammatory cells into the wound area; formation of granulation tissue; synthesis of proteins of the extracellular matrix; angiogenesis; gradual replacement of granulation tissue by connective tissue.

Chapter 4

1. 4, 2, 4, 1, 2, 14.
2. The Fab region binds antigen and comprises variable amino acid sequence. The Fc region does not interact with antigen and the amino acid sequence is constant.

3. Ten.
4. $(\gamma_2 k_2)$ or $(\gamma_2 \lambda_2)$.
5. Mature red blood cells.
6. A single B cell can produce antibody of only one antigen specificity. When Ig is being synthesized, mRNA is made from the DNA. If the DNA were not rearranged, all mRNAs could not be identical hence not all antibodies could be identical. When DNA is rearranged every Ig protein produced must have the identical peptide sequence.
7.

MHC Class I	MHC Class II
One peptide chain + β_2 microglobulin	Two peptide chains
Binds peptides of well-defined length	Binds peptides of variable lengths
Presents endogenous antigen	Presents exogenous antigen

8. CD2, CD3, CD8.
9. Immunological tolerance is a state of non-responsiveness against self antigens. It arises because all T cells bearing TCR capable of binding strongly to self MHC + self peptide are deleted during maturation in the thymus.
10. Di-sulphide bridges between adjacent cysteine residues (i.e. forming cystine).

Chapter 5

1. IgM predominates in the primary response, IgG or IgA predominate in the secondary response. In the secondary response the antibodies have a higher average affinity for antigen.
2. An intracellular virus.
3. A bacterium, fungus or yeast that has been ingested or inhaled.
4. $CD4^+$ Th1 cells.
5. CTL; IFN; phagocytosis of opsonized extracellular viruses.
6. Most antigens are T-dependent so cannot activate B cells directly. The stimulation of B cells is directed by activated T cells in an antigen-specific manner. The T cells have been selected such that they can be activated on contact with self antigens there potentially self-reactive B cells cannot be activated. All T-independent antigens are components of microorganisms.
7. APC releases IL-1; T cell expresses IL-2 receptor; T cell stimulated by IL-2; T cell releases IFNγ and MHC Class II expression upregulated on APC; T cells proliferate; memory T cells develop; T cell interacts with B cell; IL-4 produced by T cells; B cell proliferates; B cells differentiate to form antibody-secreting plasma cells.

8. Complementary pairs of molecules on T cell and APC surfaces that interact when TCR binds with MHC + antigen to strengthen adhesion between the two cell types and generate signals necessary for T cell activation. No signal is generated unless the TCR–MHC interaction takes place.

9. Antigen that enters the body orally will be presented to intraepithelial lymphocytes (IEL) and tolerance will ensue, not response. The IEL migrate between the gut lymphoid tissue and other body tissues such that the tolerance becomes systemic. If antigens that cause the response in multiple sclerosis are given orally, tolerance may be induced and so the disease process could be diminished.

10. In the lymph nodes.

Chapter 6

1. Suppressed immune responses or wounds.

2. (a) CMI; (b) Ab; (c) both.

3. Post-transplant patients need to receive immunosuppressive therapy to prevent rejection. The most frequently used drug is cyclosporin, however its dosage must be regulated carefully to avoid nephrotoxicity. It is normally metabolized by cytochrome P450 in the liver. Anti-fungal drugs inhibit P450 thereby reducing the breakdown of cyclosporin and leading to an increased risk of nephrotoxicity.

4. Infections with helminthic worms.

5. Intracellular bacteria gain entry to phagocytes or enter via phagocytosis. Most have evolved strategies to prevent their destruction by the killing mechanisms of phagocytes. They remain in the phagosomes or cytosol hidden from the cells and molecules of the immune system.

6. Antibodies are effective against extracellular viruses so many of these will be removed early in the infection. Many viruses rapidly enter host cells, predominantly $CD4^+$ T cells, where they are incorporated into the genome. They are hidden from antibodies and, because viral protein is not being made, no antigens are being presented on to activate $CD8^+$ cells.

7. In hepatitis B infection viral peptides may be displayed on Class I MHC molecules on hepatocytes. $CD8^+$ CTLs would then destroy the virally infected cells leading to liver damage and the symptoms of this severe disease. Hepatitis C virus infection leads to a chronic liver disease with little evidence of liver damage. It is likely that hepatitis C does not induce a strong CTL response.

8. The fibrin is a host molecule so the organism is not regarded as being foreign.

9. Passive immunization may induce serum sickness through the development of immune complex-mediated hypersensitivity

(Type III); the antiserum has to be re-administered on each contact with the pathogen.

10. A purified subunit vaccine is only a small part of the microorganism so there is no risk of infection. An attenuated vaccine contains the whole live microorganism but in a weakened form. Even the mild infection may be hazardous to the person with a suppressed immune response.

Chapter 7

1. The Fc portion of IgE molecules differs from other isotypes in that it contains an additional CH domain.

2. Atopy is a skin reaction that occurs in many allergic individuals when exposed to allergen.

3. $CD4^+$ Th2 cells produce IL-4 that favours switching to IgE production. Mast cells also respond to IL-4. Th2 cells also produce IL-10 that inhibits IFNγ, suppressing Th1. Excessive Th2 activity, relative to Th1, may, then, be associated with Type I hypersensitivity.

4. Anaphylactic shock involves rapid vasodilatation within the periphery. Significant volumes of blood drain from the central organs into the opened capillaries leading to consequences such as loss of consciousness. The injected adrenaline induces the characteristic 'fight or flight' response in which blood is rapidly returned from the periphery and back to the vital organs.

5. The administered anti-D, plus complement, destroys any of the baby's RBC that may have entered the mother's circulation. She does not then mount an immune response and the small amount of anti-D is rapidly cleared from her circulation.

6. When antibodies specific for the transplanted cells/tissues already exist in the recipient due to previous transplant(s) or transfusion(s).

7. Persistent exposure to low-dose antigen; low affinity antibody; complement deficiencies.

8. Dendritic cells are Langerhans cells that migrate from the tissues to lymph nodes.

9. Lepromatous leprosy involves granulomata in the skin and is associated with reduced T cell function. Tuberculoid leprosy occurs with intact T cell function and causes damage to Schwann cells of the nervous system.

10. Lipopolysaccharide (endotoxin) from the cell wall of Gram + ve bacteria is a potent stimulator of pro-inflammatory cytokines.

Chapter 8

1. Autoimmunity, the existence of autoantibodies or autoreactive T cells, is a normal, physiological finding. Autoimmune disease

is the association of apparently autoimmune mechanisms with disease symptoms.

2. Rheumatoid factor (RF) is antibody directed against self IgG; it is usually of the IgM type or, occasionally, IgG.

3. In autoimmune diseases the use of immunosuppressive drugs would lead to an improvement in symptoms; infections would become more severe. Many autoreactive cells or autoantibodies in an affected tissue would be directed against the same antigen as shown by the use of a restricted range of V region genes; in infected tissues a wide range of different epitopes, and hence V regions, would be involved.

4. IFN-β.

5. When some antigens are ingested they lead to systemic tolerance. Known autoantigens can be fed to induce tolerance and so diminish the autoimmune response.

6. A test for the detection of antibodies to double-stranded DNA.

7. An autoantibody is generated against thyroid-stimulating hormone (TSH) receptors on the thyroid gland. This stimulates the production of thyroid hormones which are unable to regulate their synthesis through the normal mechanism of TSH down-regulation. Thyroid stimulation through the autoantibody persists.

8. In MG an autoantibody binds to acetylcholine receptors (AChR) on post-synaptic neurons. Acetylcholine released into the synapse is unable to interact with the AChR so the nervous impulse is not transmitted efficiently and muscles are not stimulated.

9. When cells are placed under stress they synthesize stress proteins, e.g. HSP. Stress proteins are highly conserved through evolution so simple organisms such as bacteria express proteins that show considerable homology with human HSP. Immune responses directed against bacterial proteins may cross-react with human HSP on host cells leading to cell damage.

10. Family studies in which close relatives may have similar susceptibilities to autoimmune diseases; individuals who all express similar MHC alleles, e.g. particular ethnic groups, may have similar susceptibility to an autoimmune disease; the risk that a person carrying a particular MHC allele may develop an autoimmune disease is greater than for a person who does not express that allele.

Chapter 9

1. Common variable immunodeficiency (CVI). The other possibility is XLA, however that deficiency is inborn so would lead to recurrent infections at an early stage of life. The X-chromosome linkage of XLA would also make its occurrence rare in a female and all Ig isotypes are likely to be equally affected in XLA. On

the other hand, CVI symptoms can occur in later life; it is not X-linked and different Ig isotypes may be affected to a different extent.

2. Immunodeficiency with Hyper IgM (also called hyper-IgM syndrome).

3. IgA.

4. DiGeorge's syndrome.

5. Any mature lymphocytes in the bone marrow graft would be called passenger cells. As SCID children have no effective immune response, these T cells and B cells would begin to attack the graft recipient. This is graft-versus-host disease and is fatal.

6. NADPH oxidase. Its absence prevents effective killing of ingested organisms by phagocytes following phagocytosis.

7. Nutritional deficiencies; the presence of other illness, e.g. infections; decreased efficiency of physical barriers, e.g. skin.

8. d.

9. Anti-HIV antibodies may help to reduce the number of virus particles binding to extracellular virus thus rendering it incapable of interacting with CD4 as is necessary to infect cells. The antibodies may promote infection because phagocytes bearing Fc receptors bind to the antibody–HIV complex and ingest it.

10. The infected cells are $CD4^+$ T cells and other cells such as macrophages. All of these cell types migrate to the secondary lymphoid tissues. Infected T cells are destroyed by virus so do not appear in the circulation. Other $CD4^+$ cells are not killed but can persist in the lymphoid tissues providing a 'safe haven' for replicating virus.

Chapter 10

1. Polyclonal antibodies are the products of several different clones of B cells while monoclonal antibodies are derived from a single B cell clone. A solution of polyclonal antibodies will show specificity for a range of antigen whereas monoclonal antibodies will have a single antigen specificity.

2. Immunoassays have increased specificity, increased sensitivity and increased flexibility of test platform relative to conventional biochemical tests.

3. In the avidin–biotin complex (ABC) method a biotinylated enzyme label is pre-incubated with avidin. Each avidin molecule is a tetramer so can bind four molecules of the biotinylated enzyme. Large complexes are assembled that can then be incubated with a biotinylated antibody.

4. Indirect immunohistochemical techniques allow the amplification of a signal indicating that antibody binding has occurred. This is because several molecules of enzyme-labelled secondary antibody can bind to each primary antibody molecule. In direct

methods the label is attached to the primary antibody so this amplification step cannot occur.

5. Endogenous peroxidase activity will need to be blocked if an antibody is used that is labelled with peroxidase. When the substrate of the label is added to the tissue the endogenous enzyme could lead to product formation thereby generating a non-specific signal.

6. In a 'sandwich' ELISA an antigen is sandwiched between two identical antibodies one of which is conjugated to the solid support (microtitre well surface) with the other carrying the label. This type of assay requires that the antigen has multiple binding sites for the same antibody.

7. The possible side-effects of high-dose IL-2 infusion include: fever, diarrhoea, thrombocytopenia, pulmonary oedema, confusion, sleepiness, disorientation, depression, insomnia and coma.

8. A HAMA response is associated with the repeated in vivo administration of murine antibodies. These are recognized as being foreign so an adaptive response is mounted against them.

9. LAK cells are lymphokine activated killer cells. These are immune cells harvested from a patient that are incubated in vitro with cytokines prior to re-infusion into the patient.

10. Tumour necrosis factor α (TNF-α).

Index

Printed in the United Kingdom
by Lightning Source UK Ltd.
130522UK00001B/58/A